NICKI WILLIAMS

LIFE AFTER MENOPAUSE

EMBRACE YOUR NEXT CHAPTER WITH A HEALTHY BODY AND MIND

PRAISE FOR *LIFE AFTER MENOPAUSE*

"I love this book. Inspiring for every woman over 50. It's the ultimate guide to living optimally in your third act."
Suzy Walker, Journalist, author and founder of The Alnwick Story Fest

"Menopause affects women differently – there's no one-size-fits-all solution, so it's important to educate yourself to make informed choices. It shouldn't be seen as the start of the end; it should be the beginning of a new chapter and one you want to own for yourself."
Shaa Wasmund MBE, author of Stop Talking, Start Doing

"Nicki was one of the first nutritionists to recognise the impact of food and lifestyle on perimenopause in the UK. She has a rare ability to take the complexity of our biochemistry to make things both easy to grasp and easy to do. In Life After Menopause she is one of the first to respond to our collective need for a blueprint post menopause too. This book is rigorously researched, full of useful tools – but critically it's a rallying call to reframe ageing and embrace our bodies and minds as they age and to find our joy in Part 2."
Rebekah Brown, founder and Head of Research, LIMINAL

"This book is truly empowering. There are many books out there supporting women going through perimenopause and menopause but there is very little out there about what happens next. For anyone who is looking for sound advice and evidence-based information on how to live a longer, healthier and happier life post menopause – this book is for you!"

**Katie Taylor, menopause campaigner and founder
of the Latte Lounge**

"When I read Life After Menopause, my first thought was, 'I so wish this had been available when I stepped over the threshold'.

As a nutrition and hormone expert, Nicki wears her (extensive) knowledge lightly. Her latest book contains a wealth of sensible, effective advice on food, supplements, exercise, sleep and hormone management, underpinned by the latest research and science.

Nicki never assumes or patronises, instead warmly conveying her guidance in a way that clarifies and supports. Especially close to my heart are her messages about putting ourselves first, and the liberating opportunities and potential that can accompany this life-stage when we consciously give ourselves permission to prioritise our own needs.

If you want to boost your mental, physical and emotional health after menopause, give yourself this book as a gift, or ask someone to get it for you."

**Caroline Ferguson, mindset trainer and author of
'Something More' on Substack**

"Loved this book, informative and encouraging as one. It's made me make some easy changes in my lifestyle without making me feel guilty and because it's so well explained it makes sense. Great to have so much information in one place and very readable."
Lynva Russell, BEM and Chair of River Holme Connections

"Nicki's book is rigorously researched and well written. An invaluable reference text for well-informed navigation of what can be a bewildering phase of life."
Dr Nerina Ramlakhan, physiologist, sleep expert, author and speaker

FOREWORD

I am a proud father. My daughter Nicki has followed up her bestselling debut, It's Not You, It's Your Hormones, with another impressive offering, covering your health journey post menopause and into old age.

The book is intensively researched and expertly structured giving solace to those geeky researchers who enjoy biochemistry and physiology, as well as those women who respond better to old-fashioned advice and common sense.

Much of the advice will apply to both men and women and superbly lays out in detail how to get the full health benefits from diet, exercise, sleep, supplements, hormone restoration and stress control, with some of the latest research on longevity supplements.

As a lifelong proponent of the benefits of Bio-Identical Hormone Replacement Therapy (BHRT) and seeing the benefits to my patients in general health, disease prevention and longevity, I am glad to see that it takes some prominence in this book.

This is a book I would have been proud to have written myself but am gratified that the apples do not fall far from the tree. It's your ideal companion in your ongoing health journey both as a reference book to dip into or as a fascinating read.

Dr Bernard Willis, MBChB, MRCGP, DObstRCOG

TABLE OF CONTENTS

INTRODUCTION

A PERSONAL UPDATE

This book was never supposed to happen. I thought I had discovered all the answers about how to be healthy. It was working fine. Until it wasn't.

It's 15 years since my dad told me I was going through perimenopause (I was 42). That's when he gave me the education that I had not received in school, university or from my doctor. The kind of knowledge we all need! Like what hormones are, how they impact how we feel and how they change throughout our lives.

I had not been feeling right since I hit 40. I had two young children and a very busy corporate job, and as any woman knows, the effort to try to be good at everything is exhausting. I was tired, stressed out, moody and had terrible brain fog that was affecting my work. This wasn't me, and I didn't know how to get back to my old self.

My doctor gave me a prescription for antidepressants when I told him my symptoms. But I instinctively knew it wasn't depression. I just didn't know what it was until I phoned my dad in floods of tears! That's when he told me it was perimenopause.

I had to get some tests done to be sure (I was ever the sceptic), but the results were clear. I had to follow his advice and start looking after my hormones.

I made some changes to my diet and lifestyle and within a few weeks, my efforts were already being rewarded. My energy was coming back, my brain fog lifted, my mood more balanced and I had even started shedding a bit of my 'stress belly'.

I was amazed at the results, but more astonished that I didn't have a clue about what was happening in my own body and how to deal with it. I was lucky that I had my dad to turn to when I was struggling (and that he was a hormone doctor with 40 years' experience), but what did other women do? I was angry that they were left to struggle on alone. Things have massively improved since then, but at that time there was very little support or information for women to get the help they needed. Doctors were doling out antidepressants as first-line treatment and most had no idea about diet, lifestyle or supplements that could help.

I had to try to change things. I went on a mission to learn more and share it among as many women as possible. I believed we had suffered a huge injustice and felt compelled to make a difference. I knew this would not only improve women's lives, but the lives of everyone around them. Especially the children, the future generations to come. If I could play a small part in making that kind of difference, I'd be very happy.

After four years of re-training to qualify as a nutritionist and hormone specialist, I founded Happy Hormones for Life in 2014, and have since been supporting women (and men) to rebalance and get back in control of their hormones and health.

When I was 49, my first book, It's Not You, It's Your Hormones, was published. In it I shared my experience and the four steps I used to rebalance my hormones and get back to my best. I continue to update it, so it's still very relevant today for every woman going through perimenopause.

But if you'd told me I would write another book, I'd have said you were mad!

It took a lot out of me to write the first one. And I honestly thought that was it. I'd discovered what worked for me, and for many other women who we were supporting through our courses, testing and programmes.

But when I hit 50, things started to change. I suddenly started getting multiple hot sweats during the night that floored me. I had experienced the odd hot flush before, but nothing like this. Waking up at night dripping with sweat was not something I had expected to happen. I thought my natural solutions would keep menopausal symptoms at bay. But these night sweats were killing me. My sleep suffered. I was more tired and moody. And I was putting on weight again.

I actually felt like a fraud. Here was me, an author and so-called expert, telling women that my natural solutions were enough to ward off the worst symptoms. And it wasn't working 100% on me!

Once again I turned to my dad. Yep, he said, you're going to need some extra help. Time to consider HRT. Now I had had many clients who were doing great on HRT, and I knew that the new form of HRT (body identical) was safe and effective. I knew from my research that taking it would be beneficial for my bones, heart and brain – let alone my skin, hair, joints and vagina!

On top of that I knew that I might be at extra risk of osteoporosis as my mum had been diagnosed with it a few years earlier.

But I wanted to be sure. I did the comprehensive urine hormone test that we routinely do with our clients at Happy Hormones. Sure enough, my results showed my oestrogen and progesterone were both low. My testosterone was also on the floor. AND my cortisol levels were way lower than I wanted them to be (not too surprising as I had always struggled with my adrenals).

So I went back to my GP for the first time since my early 40s. This time I was properly informed. In fact, I was the expert in the room. My doctor didn't know the difference between synthetic and natural HRT – had no clue about the brands I was asking for (he had to look them up). But thankfully he didn't fight me and gave me what I wanted.

I started taking oestrogen gel and a progesterone capsule at night, and after a couple of days, the night sweats stopped. I also started taking a localised oestrogen pessary, which helps with vaginal dryness (more on that later).

I couldn't get testosterone from my doctor, but did manage to go privately for that. Just a small dose of cream has increased my levels to normal. Women need testosterone too! It helps with brain health, bone support, libido and drive.

Today, at 57, I'm following my four-step Happy Hormone Code (with a balanced 80/20 ratio) and I'm taking body identical HRT. It's a powerful combination, but I'm not afraid to say that I'm still a work in progress.

I have gained over a stone in weight since I hit 50. And despite trying every tool in my toolkit, plus supplements and powders that I know can help with metabolism, nothing has worked.

It's a hard one for me to admit and deal with. But I have come to a place of acceptance. If my body is fighting like hell to retain my fat stores, maybe there's a reason for that? There's so much we don't know about metabolism, especially for women in or beyond menopause.

So, I'm making peace with my fuller body for now, absolutely no point fighting it or stressing. That's only going to make it worse and add to my frustration (and cortisol!).

Instead of obsessing about my weight, I've switched my focus to getting strong and fit. It feels amazing. And I'm remembering that it's a privilege to even be my age and have no major health worries. I am so grateful for the things my body does for me every minute of every day. As my lovely friend and mindset coach Caroline Ferguson says, "Your body is your home, make sure it's the best home it can be for you."

I also still struggle with stress, which has always been my biggest hormone saboteur. Ever since my early 40s, cortisol for me has been my main imbalance. I've done many things to address it, including meditation, breath work, yoga and supplements.

However, during the Covid pandemic, my resilience, like that of many others, was truly put to the test. Our clinic was hugely busy, with twice the usual number of clients seeking our help. And while it was amazing that we could help so many more women, it was difficult to suddenly ramp up our systems and team to cope, without letting anyone down or compromising our service. After two years of 'coping' with this unexpected growth, I was exhausted, physically and mentally. So much so, that I was close to winding up the business.

Looking back now, I can't believe that I was so depleted and low that I even had those thoughts. My work is my life! It's what I spent years re-training for, and years dedicating myself to. I can't imagine doing anything else.

But that's what adrenal fatigue looks like. You're so tired and depleted that even the things you love don't bring you the joy they should.

After a lot of reflection (and time), I realised that giving up was the last thing I wanted, I just needed to take some time to slow down and replenish.

Giving myself some space to think is exactly how this book came about. What was slowly dawning on me was that my work was not done. I'd only really addressed the first stage of the menopause transition – the perimenopause. And since I wrote my first book, there are now thankfully a whole array of books on how to get through menopause.

But what happens next? Where is the inspiration and advice for women AFTER menopause? Do we just become 'old crones' and disappear into invisibility, waiting for the end? Or do we step up, reinvent ourselves, use our incredible wisdom and experience to create a new vision for this next stage of our lives? A more peaceful, balanced and healthy version of ourselves. And become positive role models to the next generation, so that they can have a healthier and happier future.

So this is Part 2 of the transition; the next chapter. Writing this now at 57, I'm done with menopause. I'm officially postmenopausal. The landscape is very different to my 40s and I'm having to use different tools to navigate this new phase.

The postmenopausal world has new and different challenges to offer us, least of all our ageing bodies. Nature may not be on our side for this stretch, but we certainly have plenty of things we can do to protect ourselves and give ourselves the best chance of a happy and healthy old age.

Time comes at us fast, but with the right tools (and a bit of luck), we've potentially got 30-plus years ahead of us. Let's make the right choices now so that we can fully EMBRACE this exciting new chapter of our lives!

Are you ready? If the answer is yes, that's amazing. I'm excited to be your guide.

If the answer is no, or not yet, then stick with me. I hope I can persuade you that this can be the very best time of your life.

HOW TO USE THIS BOOK

This is not another book about hormones or menopause (although I will be covering them both). This book is a blueprint for a more vital and healthy future, where we can thrive, not just survive. To EMBRACE this second half of our lives, fully making use of that acquired experience and wisdom to make ourselves happier, but also pass on to the next generation who really do need our help. If we do this, we'll leave a lasting legacy and leave the world a better place.

Whether you are postmenopausal naturally (typically occurring in your early 50s), prematurely (primary ovarian insufficiency), surgically (through ovary removal), or through the effects of medical treatment, you have been through a massive upheaval. And ahead is a brand-new landscape that you may need some new tools to navigate.

And if you're still in perimenopause (still having periods), then this book will help you navigate through your menopause and get you out the other side thriving and ready for the next stage of your life. I would also recommend you get my previous book It's Not You, It's Your Hormones to give you the toolkit for this specific stage.

I'm not a doctor (or life coach) and nothing in this book constitutes medical advice, however I am a nutritionist, trained in the Functional Medicine approach, which looks at the body as an integrated, interconnected web of systems and communication.

And I'm a living human being going through it all myself the best I can.

In this book, I'm using my knowledge and clinical experience from the last ten years running my Happy Hormones clinic, along with new research and resources, to give you my best tips and recommendations on how to look after your physical and emotional health as you get older.

None of this is universal truth and not all of it will work for everyone. I'm certainly not telling you to do what I do, but I will show you what the scientific research is saying has health benefits. From there, you must work out what works for you, your body and your lifestyle.

Throughout your life, your physical and emotional health is influenced by all sorts of things – your unique genetic blueprint, your past experiences, your diet, lifestyle, stress levels, mindset, emotions, environment and also what else is going on in your body.

This all makes every woman's journey through midlife a totally unique one.

For this reason, there is no one-size-fits-all solution, no magic pill, therapy or protocol. And it's also why you'll see a myriad of different approaches to midlife challenges from a multitude of different experts, many offering their solution as the 'only' solution.

I prefer to approach wellbeing as more of a jigsaw puzzle. It can be complex and multifaceted, with many different pieces that need to be put together to form the bigger picture of optimal health and happiness. It's important to recognise that your body, mind and spirit are all interconnected and deeply impact your health and wellbeing.

Your jigsaw picture is going to be different to anyone else's. You are totally unique, with your own individual gene expressions, diets, lifestyles, beliefs, emotions, stresses, backgrounds, circumstances, relationships, mindset, support, resilience, influences and even unique ways your body works.

In this book, I am giving you lots of options. Choose what feels good for you and create your own personalised toolkit – whether that involves seeking medical advice, making lifestyle changes such as improving nutrition and exercise habits, or seeking support from friends, family, or professionals to help with emotional health, transitions or mindset.

But certainly don't try to do it all, and definitely don't let anything in this book cause you added worry or stress. If you need to, use this opportunity to create the space and time to sit in the mud for a while, embracing uncertainty, while you slowly work out what your needs are and what the rest of your life might look like if you met them fully (and maybe for the first time). That's fine too.

In Part 1 we explore the new landscape of life after menopause. We look at our lifespan versus health span and how to make the most of our extending life expectancy by living well and not just longer. We look at the stigma of ageing and all our modern-day challenges. And we flip the old negative paradigm of ageing and get excited about the huge possibilities of this next phase of our lives. We'll also cover the science of the ageing process, physically and psychologically.

Part 2 looks at how you're feeling post menopause - physically and emotionally. What's going on for you? You can dip in and out of this one according to your own symptoms. This section covers some common health symptoms, the possible causes and some key tips to help you overcome them and start feeling better.

Part 3 is all about how to EMBRACE life after menopause. We will look at the EMBRACE protocol of healthy ageing to get you thinking about and planning your personal journey ahead to the most healthy, happy and vibrant YOU post menopause.

I'll also be including stories of some of the amazing inspirational women over 50 that I've met in my time at Happy Hormones, some of whom I've interviewed for my podcast.

RESOURCES AND REFERENCES

Throughout my research for this book, I have discovered numerous wonderful organisations and resources that may be helpful for your health journey. In the Resources section, you'll find a curated list of books and websites to explore further.

I have created a workbook to accompany this book, which will help you create your own personal plan. You can download the online version at www.happyhormonesforlife.com/life. You can also purchase a print version if you prefer.

This book is grounded in respected scientific literature, with numerous references to support the information presented. To save paper, I have compiled all references and links on my website.

www.happyhormonesforlife.com/life
or scan the QR code below

STATEMENT AND DISCLAIMERS

Inclusivity statement:

In this book, I will be using the terms 'woman' and 'women' when discussing female hormones, menopause and other health issues. However, I want to make it clear that I am doing so inclusively, referring to all people who may be affected by these issues. My aim is to create a safe and welcoming space for all readers, regardless of their gender identity or health status, and to provide valuable information and support for anyone who is navigating the challenges of life after menopause.

Medical disclaimer:

The information presented in this book is for informational purposes only and is not intended as a substitute for advice from your physician or doctor or other health care professional. You should consult with a physician, doctor or health care professional before undertaking any diet, exercise or supplement programme, before taking any medication or nutritional supplement, or if you have or suspect you might have a health problem. The author and publishers cannot be held responsible for any errors and omissions that may be found in the text or any actions that may be taken by a reader as a result of any reliance on the information contained in the text, which is taken entirely at the reader's own risk.

Now the formalities are done with, let's get started …

PART 1

THE NEXT CHAPTER:

Challenges and Opportunities

CHAPTER 1

LIVING BETTER, NOT JUST LONGER

Welcome to life after menopause!

Let's take a moment to check in. How are you feeling? No, really feeling? Has your menopause transition been a smooth meander down the river or more of a wild ride down the rapids?

Menopause can be brutal. Physically and emotionally.

You may have stepped off the crazy perimenopause roller coaster, but your body is no doubt still adapting to a new hormonal status with either lingering symptoms or brand-new ones to deal with.

And your emotions might still be reeling as you come to terms with your changing body and any midlife transitions you may be going through.

The good news is that you're coming out the other side. And with that you have an opportunity to start designing a life that will bring you more joy, vitality and fulfilment.

And we've got time on our side if we get this right. Beyond menopause, we're living longer than ever.

According to data from the Society of Actuaries, a 45-year-old woman today who is a non-smoker and describes her health as excellent has a greater than 50% likelihood of reaching age 90, a 37% chance of reaching age 95, and close to a 20% chance of reaching age 100.

That means that although the average life expectancy for a woman born today in the UK is just shy of 83, it's quite likely that 1 in 5 of you reading this will reach 100.

For many of us, this is a time that's unmapped and uncharted. A huge opportunity to fully enjoy the advantages of longevity, such as wisdom, freedom, resilience and experience. It's a chance to reinvent our lives, reach our potential, enjoy ourselves and to put our needs FIRST for once.

Unfortunately it's harder to do that if we're not physically and mentally well. And the stats are not encouraging.

According to the McKinsey Health Institute, global life expectancy has more than doubled in the last 200 years, but the proportion of life spent in poor or moderate health remains at 50%. This means half of our lives are spent in poor health, and this issue isn't limited to lower-income countries.

In the UK, the Health Foundation's 2023 report projects that nearly 1 in 5 people will have a major illness by 2040, an increase of over a third from current levels. They state, "chronic conditions now afflict growing numbers of people for a significant portion of their lives."

Women, despite living six years longer on average than men, often experience more health issues. Dr Libby Weaver, in her book *Rushing Woman Syndrome*, notes that we are "living too short and dying too long," with many facing years of chronic pain, multiple medications and medical care needs.

The good news is that how we live can improve our 'health span' – the number of years we live in good health and – and help maximise the years ahead.

CHAPTER 2

REFRAMING AGEING

AGEISM

We can't discuss ageing without exploring the impact of society's perception of the older woman. Ageism, a discrimination based on age, hits women particularly hard, compounding the challenges they've already faced from gender bias throughout their lives.

Let's just firstly reflect on how entrenched gender bias is before we tackle ageing stereotypes for women. The United Nations Development Programme issued a report in 2023 that really stunned me. The study captured people's attitudes globally on women's roles in different aspects of society.

Shockingly the results showed that almost 9 out of 10 people (of all genders) thought men were better than women – in the workplace, in politics, in education and pretty much every area of life (including 25% of people thinking it's justifiable for a man to beat his wife). Bearing in mind these were global perspectives, including those from lower-income countries, the most alarming thing is that this figure hasn't changed in a decade.

With this sobering backdrop in mind, let's delve into the attitudes surrounding ageing women.

Ashton Applewhite (author of *This Chair Rocks*) explains how early ageist agendas start. As young girls we are drip fed that ageing is bad, that youth is everything and so by the time we are in our 20s and 30s we are already afraid of every new wrinkle, line or that very first grey hair! Young women are having Botox in their 20s, using anti-wrinkle creams, and staying out of the sun to avoid skin damage (I'm not saying that's not sensible, but we do need vitamin D too!).

Our Western patriarchal societal attitudes towards older women are awful. Instead of revering older women for their wisdom and experience, they are often ignored, pushed aside, perceived as ugly, useless, irrelevant or just plain invisible. Old age is seen as a time of loss and decay, waiting for the final curtain.

By contrast, in traditional cultures, such as the Mayans, Māoris and Iroquois, menopause holds a special significance for women as a powerful transition. It's a time when women step into their deepest feminine power, gaining a newfound status as wise leaders and role models. This transformative phase allows them to share the wealth of knowledge and wisdom they have accumulated throughout their lives, benefiting not only themselves but also the entire tribe. They are seen as 'elders' not 'elderly'.

In ancient times, words like 'crone' and 'hag' were used to celebrate older women. Being called a 'crone' meant you were a wise and respected woman, someone whose wisdom was highly valued. And the word 'hag' actually comes from 'hagio', which means holy. But no woman wants these labels today!

According to GenM's UK Menopause Market Report in 2023, more women than ever are feeling 'invisible', 'lonely', 'dispensable' or 'irrelevant'. The report says that "while menopause is a shared experience, it is becoming increasingly isolating for many". Over half the women surveyed felt unattractive and lacked confidence.

They go on to say that "society views women as invisible and dried up after their fertility stops, but this isn't the case. It shouldn't be viewed as an illness."

Big businesses fuel the negative narrative around ageing by playing on our insecurities. Cosmetics, creams and supplements aimed at holding onto your youth are hugely lucrative. We are made to feel ashamed by our imperfections, less attractive if we look older. And that brings up deep primal fears of being abandoned, rejected, unloved, useless and alone. No wonder we try so hard to look younger!

Career-wise, women over 50 are the fastest growing workforce demographic, yet ageist perceptions hinder their access to the best jobs, equal pay, training and advancement opportunities. Women often feel they are held to higher standards than their male counterparts at work, so have to work harder to prove themselves. Not surprisingly, more women are burning out and quitting their careers.

Gender and age bias have deep and long-lasting roots within the field of health and medicine. From limited research on women's health concerns, particularly as they age, to disparities in the diagnosis and treatment of medical conditions, traditional medicine and research has been male-focused for generations. There is clear underrepresentation of older women in clinical trials, and older women face systemic barriers to accessing healthcare services and often encounter dismissive attitudes from healthcare providers (as well as my own personal experience, I hear stories of this every day from women).

If you type 'postmenopausal women' into Google images, you'll likely encounter a lot of white, grey-haired women with head in hands, having a hot flush, or looking miserable! And the impact of all this is profound, not only on our health outcomes but also on our overall happiness as we journey through the years. Especially if you don't see yourself represented in these images (e.g. if you're from an ethnic minority, and/or the trans or non-binary communities).

When we face ageist attitudes and stereotypes, it can significantly affect our mental health. Self-esteem can take a big hit, and we're more likely to struggle with things like depression and anxiety. It's like a vicious cycle, we can start believing we're not as capable or worthy just because of our age.

And let's not forget about the physical effects. Ageism-induced stress is a real problem. It can increase the risk of cardiovascular disease, cognitive decline, and even shorten our lifespan. And to make things worse, as women, we risk not getting the best attention or treatment we need from the medical establishment.

But we don't have to sit down and accept this! Let's tackle these out of date and ridiculous attitudes about older women. Because here's the truth: these stereotypes couldn't be further from reality. Older women are a vibrant and diverse group, brimming with wisdom, resilience and vitality.

In fact, in 2024's Forbes 100 Most Powerful Women list, 80% of them were over 50! I'd love you to take inspiration from them and the amazing women I highlight in this book, along with iconic older figures like Julia Roberts, Oprah, Gillian Anderson, Prue Leith, Iman, Jane Fonda, Helen Mirren, Nigella Lawson, Viola Davis and many other amazing women that are over 50 and full of vitality.

Let's rewrite the narrative, break down old attitudes and redefine what it means to age with grace and strength. We deserve to be seen, heard and celebrated for our invaluable contributions to society.

The wisdom of menopausal women is vital for community survival, and the more we celebrate this, the more we can change the cultural paradigm, empower ourselves and others, command respect, and be powerful role models to inspire the next generation.

POSITIVE AGEING

Your Mind
Are you a natural optimist or pessimist? Glass half full or half empty?

It might seem obvious that your diet and lifestyle has an impact on how well you age, but did you know that how you think about life and ageing can not only affect your happiness and satisfaction with life, but it can also help you live longer?

We know from research that how you think and feel about the menopause can affect how severe your symptoms are. One cross-cultural review of menopause experiences globally concluded that, "Menopausal symptoms seem to be caused by a combination of physical changes, cultural influences, and individual perceptions and expectations."

It's no coincidence that in Japan, the word for menopause is *konenki*, literally meaning 'renewal of years' or 'change of seasons', a much more exciting description than just 'men' (month) and 'pause' (stopping), which is rather less inspiring!

Mayan women that still reside in Central and South America have been interviewed about their menopause experiences. Regardless of whether they experienced symptoms or not, they seemed to look forward to menopause, viewing it as a time of newfound freedom and elevated status as they became spiritual leaders within their communities.

Beyond menopause, it's been shown that a positive outlook on ageing can potentially extend your life by a whopping eight years compared to someone with more negative perspectives, and more importantly, increase your happiness in those years. The researchers concluded that, "Self-perceptions of ageing had a greater impact on survival than did gender, socioeconomic status, loneliness and functional health."

As well as lower rates of chronic diseases, improved cognitive function, and better overall physical functioning, a positive outlook is better for your mental health.

We will discover in this book how your thoughts can affect your own physiology, with positive ones creating 'happy hormones' and negative ones creating stress hormones and inflammation. And how these thoughts and beliefs can actually influence your DNA and gene expression, and therefore your health and life expectancy.

And if you feel negativity or worry about ageing itself, you are more likely to be depressed or anxious, and engage in unhealthy behaviours such as smoking, drinking and to have poor eating and exercise habits. Definitely a vicious cycle.

The great news is that we can control and reframe our attitudes and thoughts about ageing. Have a look at some of the incredible women over 50 I've included throughout this book (Inspirational Women) who are redefining what's possible for older women.

And let's remember what we've got to feel positive about. By our 50s, we've gained a huge amount of valuable experience. We survived our troublesome teens, that awkward transition from childhood to adulthood. We're past our uncertain 20s, struggling to work out our path and who we are. We're through our 'settle down' 30s, where we were busy implementing our plan (or still winging it), and then our juggling 40s, no doubt spinning the many plates that we've thrown into the air.

What's up next for you can be either depressing and problematic OR it can be exciting and inspiring. And that of course depends on your individual circumstances, but mainly your mindset and how you deal with stress.

A positive outlook is going to produce better social connections and relationships (positivity tends to attract others), which can lead to more personal growth, self-fulfilment and a greater sense of purpose. The opposite of a vicious cycle, this is a 'virtuous cycle' or 'positive feedback loop' that breeds more positive outcomes in your life.

Who says we have to give up or slow down as we age? Carl Honoré, author of *Bolder: making the most of our longer lives* says: "We can tear up the old script that locks us into learning in early life, working in the middle years and pursuing leisure with whatever time is left at the end. Instead, we can learn, work, rest, care for others, volunteer, create and have fun all the way through our lives."

Feminist activist Gloria Steinem is attributed to saying, "We don't grow better or worse with age, just more like the unique selves we were born to be."

In her groundbreaking book *Upgrade*, Dr Louann Brizendine changes the paradigm around older women. She believes the female brain gets stronger and better in midlife and beyond! In the very first chapter, she says: "This phase is an opportunity to grow into the wisdom and strength and resilience we've been primed for across our lifespan ... Freedom from the reproductive phase is an amazing, extraordinary and now much longer period of a woman's life than ever."

It makes me think that we should not consider ageing as a *failing*, but as a fabulous sign that we are *living!*

Jane Fonda in her TED talk from 2011 talks about how the 'third act' of our lives can have its own developmental significance. And we should be asking ourselves what we want from this extra time. Jane believes that ageing should be reframed as a "staircase, an upward ascension of the human spirit, bringing us into wisdom, wholeness and authenticity". And this can happen in spite of our ageing physical bodies. How wonderful!

Cameron Diaz stated in an interview in 2014 "I always want to be changing and I always want to be getting older. I always want to be getting wise. That, to me, is a privilege."

Oprah Winfrey said: "So many women I've talked to see menopause as an ending. But I've discovered this is your moment to reinvent yourself after years of focusing on the needs of everyone else. It's your opportunity to get clear about what matters most to you and then to pursue that with all your energy, time and talent."

Helen Mirren speaks openly about ageing. She says in an

interview with Women's Health magazine, "It's great to get older, it's fantastic! You learn that it becomes less about yourself, and more about the wider world. Because it's either you die young, or you get old. And I don't want to die young: I'm too interested in life."

In Brene Brown's excellent blog, she writes, "Midlife is when the universe gently places her hands upon your shoulders, pulls you close, and whispers in your ear: *I'm not screwing around … Time is growing short. There are unexplored adventures ahead of you. You can't live the rest of your life worried about what other people think. You were born worthy of love and belonging. Courage and daring are coursing through your veins. You were made to live and love with your whole heart. It's time to show up and be seen.*"

In 2023, Caitlin Moran wrote in *The Times*, "Men's midlife crises involve a motorbike, a tattoo or remarrying … Women, however, unable to repeat their second act because their fertility has ended, have to work out a new third act. Physically and emotionally, we are something else and so our third acts tend to see the formation of entirely new lives. We get into hillwalking. We found charities. We start meditating. We garden. We get PhDs. We learn to tango. We start our own businesses. We get involved in campaigning. We buy a lot of wind chimes and put them up in the garden, despite the fact the neighbours hate them …"

In her book *The Menopausal Brain,* Dr Lisa Mosconi writes that once through the turbulence of perimenopause, women commonly report improved mood, increased patience and reduced tension, highlighting a general trend towards greater life satisfaction after menopause. She calls it 'menostart', a new adulthood or 'renaissance', marked by well-earned confidence, renewed interests, priorities and attitudes. She also explains the positive neurological changes accompanying menopause, such as enhanced emotional control and deeper empathy, which contribute to a more confident, empowered and emotionally balanced state.

A poll commissioned by UK-based food supplement company Vitabiotics of 1,000 women who are currently or have been through the menopause, found that while it is often seen as a challenge, 34% never felt 'freer' than when it was all over.

Let's flip 'anti' ageing to 'pro' ageing and focus on the benefits and positive side of getting older:

1. No more periods or monthly cycle hell!
2. Time and money saved not needing sanitary products.
3. No more worries about unwanted pregnancies.
4. Say goodbye to unwanted catcalls, comments or lustful stares as you walk down the street.
5. Enjoy the stability that comes with balanced hormones,
6. Feel liberated and unrestricted as you embrace the newfound freedom of menopause.
7. Care less about others' opinions and live life the way you want (create a 'F**kit List!).
8. Be proud; all that life experience has made you wise, strong and resilient as hell.
9. Be grateful; you're here when others may not have been so lucky.
10. Take the opportunity to create a new purpose for your life – what do you want to do with the next few decades?
11. Care less about how you look, and more about how you feel.
12. Shift the focus to your own needs and desires, prioritising self-care and self-fulfilment.

As postmenopausal women we have so much to offer. We are wiser, stronger, more independent and less fearful. And the best thing is, we are less likely to give a f**k about what other people think. That's powerful!

Your Body

A positive reframe of getting older is clearly a vital tool that not only keeps us happy as we age, but also has a positive impact on our physical health. However, mindset alone isn't enough to keep us in top shape for as long as possible.

We also have to focus on our physical health, so that we can make the most of the next chapter and live well into our old age.

Ageing or 'anti-ageing' for women has always been about beauty and aesthetics. Cosmetic surgery, Botox, fillers, liposuction and a myriad of other treatments aimed at making you 'look' younger.

While I'm not judging anyone who has this approach (I want to look my best as much as anyone else), if we don't focus on what's going on under the surface and make sure we're doing our best to age well on the inside, then it won't matter what we look like. What's the point of looking young if you're sick or can't do the things you want?

'Healthy ageing' is all about what's going on inside your body. It's the foundation of positive ageing. And it will do way more for you than just 'fixing' the way you look on the outside.

Let's long for a vibrant healthy body rather than an unrealistic skinny unblemished ideal that doesn't bring us joy. Let's not worry about what we look like in a bikini, let's focus on strength, balance, mobility, heart health, happy joints and bones, sex drive, brain health, sleep, energy, happiness, connection and a healthy gut and immune system.

The process of ageing is completely natural of course. We can't cheat it, no matter what we do. Our bodies aren't designed to last forever. Over time, they start getting less efficient at the processes that keep us alive: cell regeneration, repair, detoxification, energy production, digestion, immunity, movement, circulation of blood and nutrients and more.

All of which results in the classic signs of ageing that we will all experience.

While we can't stop our bodies chronologically ageing, the good news is that we can control how well we age through how we live.

You only have to look at studies of the five Blue Zones, where the world's oldest communities live. These are villages in Okinawa, Japan; Sardinia, Italy; Nicoya, Costa Rica; Loma Linda, California; and Icaria, Greece. People here are ten times more likely to reach the age of 100 than anywhere else.

Even though they live in very different places worldwide, they share similar health-promoting principles in their diet and lifestyle: a natural non-processed diet, daily physical activity, strong community relationships and family values, a sense of purpose and a spiritual connection.

In fact, Dan Buettner, who did much of the research on the Blue Zones concluded that the same things that help us live a long healthy life are the things that make life worth living. And you'll notice it's not just one thing that makes the difference. It's a combination of factors that will ultimately determine how well we live (and die).

We can't all live exactly like they do, but there's certainly a lot to learn from these communities. We know that obvious things like not smoking, exercising and staying at a healthy weight can increase your chance of a healthier longer life.

But what if we did more?

If we give our bodies what they need to repair cells, calm inflammation, balance hormones, feed the brain, support our bodily systems, we can seriously reduce the risk of things going wrong and suffering disease.

As well as looking after our physical health, what if we really tapped into our emotional needs too? We know that our mental and physical health is totally connected. And the evidence shows that our thoughts, emotions and mindset can dramatically affect our health outcomes.

The choices we make day to day can not only impact how we feel now, but can impact how we age in the future. We'll come to that in Part 3!

And while it's obviously better to start looking after yourself as early as possible (prevention is always easier than cure), it doesn't matter. You can start right now. However old you are, whatever your life circumstances, it's never too late to make some changes that could make a difference to your future. Even if you start small and make baby steps, you are taking action and moving towards a healthier future.

Longevity is a booming industry. Business and consumers are spending billions in the drive to live longer, healthier lives. From dietary strategies to high-tech clinics, sophisticated health tracking, biohacking and epigenetics, science is advancing, and new discoveries are being made every day.

There's even a longevity competition! It's called the Rejuvenation Olympics, where 1,750 people strive to get the largest age reversal scores. You might think this would be only for the big players like Bryan Johnson (he spends $2m a year on reversing ageing). But what's encouraging is that just below him on the scoreboard is Julie Gibson Clark, a 55-year-old whose regimen includes regular exercise, three sauna sessions per week, meditation, a diet rich in vegetables, and approximately £60 spent monthly on supplements. Her rate of ageing is 0.65 years for each additional chronological year, slightly lower than Johnson's 0.69 (normal ageing is one year per year).

What does all this mean for you and me? It means we have never had so much amazing cutting-edge information and resources available to us. We don't have to adopt extreme behaviours or spend millions, but we can learn from those that are doing just that and take what might work for us in our day-to-day lives.

For me, longevity isn't about stopping the clock, but rather enriching the time we have left. The great news for modern women is that we have choices. We have access to the best that medicine has to offer in the form of HRT and other medications if we need them, as well as a vast range of natural solutions to support us. And if we can reframe our perception of ageing through our postmenopausal era, we can embrace this new phase and make it our most exciting yet.

CHAPTER 3

THE AGEING PROCESS

There's no doubt that once we reach the middle section of our life, there are new challenges that we may be facing. Midlife and menopause can bring profound changes to your body. And the brutal truth is that ageing accelerates exponentially after 40. Menopause itself accelerates cellular ageing by 6%, according to researchers at UCLA in the US.

We are all going to age differently, but you'll have a version of these obvious signs. Your eyesight is getting worse every year. Your hair is greyer or coarser. Your body and muscles ache just getting out of bed. You forget your words, phone, keys. You stand in a room wondering why you went in there. Your skin is sagging and no amount of anti-wrinkle cream is fixing those lines. You stare at the ceiling at night worrying about not sleeping. Your weight is creeping up no matter what you eat or how much you exercise. If you're still able to cope with alcohol, the hangovers are starting to feel like it's not worth it. And your libido seems to have forgotten you exist …

These are the realities of physical ageing for many people. It can be a strange feeling, like you've got the body of an old person, when you still feel 25 in your head!

And then there's the midlife juggle. It's real, alright. Once you've done your work, got your exercise in, gone food shopping, fed yourself and anyone else you're in charge of, cleaned up, looked after kids/parents if you have them, caught up with friends/partner, run your errands, there's not much energy left for much else, let alone self-care!

No wonder we reach for that glass of wine, and most likely fall asleep on the sofa watching Netflix.

These are typical realities of psychological ageing, a mixture of emotional status, stress, environment, circumstances and relationships.

Now this may not be what's going on for you. And I really hope that you're doing well. But I do know these are some of the most common complaints from the midlife women we've seen over the years in our clinic.

On top of all that, we face some pretty scary health risks. Once we get past menopause, the risk of serious health conditions makes depressing reading. We can't hide under the duvet though, let's face this head on, then make a commitment to minimising our risk as much as possible.

Main health risks after menopause

- **Heart disease:** Cardiovascular disease is five times more likely to kill you after menopause than anything else. And it's often asymptomatic.
- **Stroke:** Women are more likely than men to have a stroke, and the risk increases after menopause. High blood pressure, high cholesterol, smoking and a family history of stroke are all risk factors.
- **Diabetes:** Postmenopausal women are at increased risk of developing type 2 diabetes, which often starts with insulin resistance.
- **Cancer:** Women are at increased risk of developing several types of cancer after menopause, including lung, breast, ovarian and uterine cancer. In fact, lung cancer is one of the leading causes of cancer-related deaths in women. Risk factors include smoking, occupation, family history and pollution.

> - **Osteoporosis:** Worldwide 1 in 3 women over 50 will suffer an osteoporotic fracture and over 60% of all fractures occur in women, usually in the hip, ankle or wrist. Osteoporosis is a condition characterised by low bone mass and deterioration of bone tissue.

OK, that's the bad news faced. The good news is that even though our health risks obviously increase as we get older, there's lots we can do to control and minimise them.

EPIGENETICS

Your genes may load the gun, but your environment pulls the trigger.

Let's face it, you're less likely to be excited about getting older if you've got a history of illness or disease in your family, and you think you're probably headed for the same outcome.

The good news is that your genes don't tell the whole story.

In fact, genes are thought to be responsible for only around 10–20% of what we see as age-related symptoms. The other 80–90% is thought to be down to your diet, lifestyle, environment and emotional health (often referred to as your 'exposome') – which means that we can have a huge impact on our health outcomes through the choices we make.

This is the nature of 'epigenetics' – the science of gene expression. Genes can be switched on and off (expressed) according to our external and internal environments.

In our external environment, we can make dietary and lifestyle choices that help to deactivate genes that promote disease while activating those that support health and longevity. Nutrigenomics is a science helping us learn more about how our individual genetic variations (Single Nucleotide Polymorphisms or SNPs) can influence the body's response to nutrients and dietary patterns. You can now test your DNA for things like fat and carbohydrate metabolism, heart and bone health, detoxification, insulin sensitivity and inflammation.

Similarly, within our internal environment, practices like stress management, meditation and positive thoughts and emotions offer the same potential to influence healthy gene expression.

And then there's something called methylation. This is a vital piece in determining how your genes are expressed. Methyl groups of chemicals attach to your DNA and control their function (activating or silencing the gene). And this process is highly influenced by you (whether you know it or not!), through your diet, lifestyle, emotions and environment. We'll look at how to positively influence methylation in Part 3.

The bottom line is that even if you have an inherited genetic condition, how you live might influence the severity of your symptoms and prognosis. And if you have a genetic susceptibility in your family history, like heart disease or cancer, or you have genetic SNPs that increase your risk of certain conditions, it doesn't have to be your destiny. If we are in control of the conditions, we can also control our gene expression by creating the right environment that helps to switch them on or off.

PHYSICAL AGEING

Before we get to how we can help ourselves stay healthy post menopause, let's explore some of the complex biological processes that contribute to physical ageing.

DNA damage

As we age, damage to our DNA becomes more common and can accelerate the ageing process. In fact, our DNA can sustain up to 100,000 hits every day due to various internal and external factors, and while our built-in repair systems can fix most of the damage, even 1% that is not repaired can accumulate over time.

We can reduce or eliminate sources of DNA-damaging insults,

such as processed foods, environmental toxins and UV radiation, and by activating our DNA repair systems, we can slow down the ageing process and reduce our risk of disease.

Senescence

Ageing isn't just about getting more aches, pains and wrinkles. What's happening under the surface in your cells is something called senescence. It's when cells stop dividing and get stuck in a kind of 'sleep mode' that they can't wake up from. These cells are often called 'zombie cells' because they're not quite alive and not quite dead, just like the fictional zombies in stories. They are the opposite of stem cells, which can self-renew, and they act differently to normal cells.

Zombie cells send out signals into their environment. Some of these signals are helpful, like stopping damaged cells from turning into cancer. But, if too many cells become senescent and keep sending out these signals, it can lead to inflammation and damage to tissues and organs, accelerating ageing and increasing the risk of chronic disease.

Senescence happens due to varying factors such as DNA damage, oxidative stress or just wear and tear. We can't stop it, but we can have an influence over how fast it happens by adopting a healthy diet and lifestyle.

Dysregulated nutrient signalling

Our intricate biological systems have developed nutrient-sensing pathways crucial for understanding how our dietary choices impact disease prevention, overall health and longevity.

However, as we age, these pathways often become dysregulated. Some become less responsive to nutrients, contributing to issues like insulin resistance, while others remain overly activated, leading to decreased cellular maintenance, increased damage and accelerated ageing. This process is further exacerbated by poor diet and lifestyle choices.

Key nutrient sensing pathways include:

- Insulin signalling (IGF-1) – insulin-like growth factor is responsible for cell growth, repair and maintenance, as well as metabolism and energy balance.
- mTOR – a protein that regulates cell growth, cell proliferation, and cell survival.
- AMPK – an enzyme that plays a role in cellular energy, metabolic health, insulin sensitivity and weight management.
- Sirtuins – a family of proteins that regulate cellular health and are involved in cellular repair, metabolism, and longevity.

We'll explore how to protect these pathways in Part 3.

Faulty proteins

Proteins serve as the foundational components and vital workers within our cells, with each cell housing millions of them. Their function is determined not only by the different amino acids they contain, but also by their shape. These proteins undergo a constant cycle of breakdown and renewal. And they can be easily damaged (just like DNA) or misshapen through ageing, diet, lifestyle and toxins.

If they are not cleared up or recycled, these faulty proteins can start to clump together and accumulate, increasing the risk of all kinds of chronic conditions. This is where autophagy comes in …

Impaired autophagy

Autophagy literally means 'self-eating', and it's a process our bodies use to detox and eliminate damaged 'stuff' inside our cells. It's essentially a recycling and disposal machine for our cellular rubbish! But as we get older, autophagy starts to slack off, meaning our cellular junk like messed-up organelles, wonky proteins and tired mitochondria can pile up, causing cells to act wonky too.

This build-up leads to problems like more oxidative stress, inflammation and cells not renewing themselves properly. Autophagy plays a role in preventing the accumulation of those senescent 'zombie' cells that trigger inflammation and reduce overall cellular performance.

The good news is that there are ways to kick autophagy back into gear so that we can age a little bit slower.

Telomere shortening

Did you know that you have little timekeepers in your cells called telomeres? Telomeres are a collection of DNA that fit like a little cap on the end of your chromosomes (a bit like the cap on the end of your shoelace).

And they shorten (or fray) as we age. Eventually they aren't able to hold the DNA inside, so they can unravel, and the cell either stops replicating or dies. Or worse, turns into one of those zombie cells, which can cause inflammation and general havoc!

Unfortunately, it looks like menopause has a role in this too. Studies have shown that a decline in oestrogen levels can cause a more rapid rate of telomere shortening.

Telomeres don't last forever, it's a normal part of ageing, but the longer we are able to keep them intact, the longer our cells are able to divide (and keep us alive).

Fortunately, we can have an impact on our own telomeres and cell health by how we live. Restoring oestrogen levels through HRT has been shown to slow down the rate of telomere shortening. We can also look after the enzyme 'telomerase' as this helps keep telomeres long. That involves managing stress, getting enough antioxidants and omega-3s in your diet, exercising and having good levels of vitamin D. We'll cover all of these in Part 3.

Faulty mitochondria

Imagine every cell in your body containing little battery packs. These are your mitochondria, tiny sausage-shaped organelles that live inside your cells. Their main job is to convert the nutrients from the food you eat into energy in the form of a molecule called ATP (adenosine triphosphate). This energy is what powers all the functions of your body, from the beating of your heart to the firing of your neurons.

The problem is that this amazingly complex process is susceptible to damage – especially as we age, but also as a result of our daily lifestyles. Mitochondria can be damaged by eating too much sugar, losing muscle mass, exposure to environmental toxins, too much stress, poor gut health, infections, inflammatory conditions and just getting older. Damaged mitochondria stimulate inflammation and harm healthy cells.

The number and condition of our mitochondria can vary greatly, resulting in differences in energy levels and overall health throughout our lifespan. Essentially, the more numerous and healthier our mitochondria are, the more energy we have and the better we feel.

Once more, there seems to be a link between mitochondrial health and sex hormone decline post menopause. Studies have shown that lower oestrogen levels after menopause can have a negative impact on mitochondrial function, leading to a decrease in energy production and an increase in oxidative stress.

However, there are ways to help support our mitochondria and make them work better. We'll be addressing this in Part 3.

Oxidation – getting rusty

One of the main drivers of ageing is a process called 'oxidation'. It's a bit like what happens to metal when it rusts. Or when an apple or avocado goes brown once it's cut into.

This also happens to our bodies. You'll see it most obviously in your skin (pigmentation, lines, sun damage, etc.), as that's the visible process happening, but it's also a natural process inside your body.

Oxidation is a chemical reaction that results in the production of free radicals. It's a very normal process and as long as we have enough antioxidants available, it won't cause too much damage. If we don't have enough antioxidants, that's when things can get out of control, and we are at increased risk of degenerative disease.

And again, we're at a disadvantage post menopause. Oestrogen is apparently an antioxidant, so it helps protect cells from oxidative damage. There's a direct link between low oestrogen levels and more oxidative stress.

Luckily we have our own inbuilt antioxidant fighter. The NRF2 pathway is a vital defence mechanism within cells, activating antioxidant and detoxification genes to combat oxidative stress and eliminate toxins. It helps maintain cellular health by neutralising reactive oxygen species and facilitating the removal of harmful compounds.

As we age, this pathway gets less efficient and dysregulation of NRF2 signalling is linked to diseases like cancer and neurodegenerative disorders.

This is where our diet can come to the rescue. Antioxidants can top up our defences, preventing or slowing down the damage that free radicals can cause. By upping our intake of antioxidants in our diet and supplements (including broccoli and green tea which are NRF2 activators), we can make sure we're on the right side of this particular battle!

Inflamm-aging

Inflammation is a normal (and vital) immune response to injury or infection. Inflamm-aging is the concept of chronic low-grade inflammation that makes us age faster.

Let's say you've just accidentally cut yourself. Your immune system rushes white blood cells, antibodies and other immune molecules to the affected site where they isolate the injury and seal off the wound to slow blood loss and ward off infection.

This process causes the area to become inflamed, which can cause redness, warmth and swelling.

More immune agents then come along to clean up the debris and prevent infection. And over time, as the wound heals, the inflammation will start to subside.

Once the crisis is averted, a healthy immune system then goes back to normal and shuts off the alarm. But when your immune system isn't at its best, it can keep the inflammation going, and if unchecked this can lead to health conditions such as diabetes, obesity, heart disease and cancer.

On top of that your immune system can start to 'misfire', to attack things that are actually harmless (e.g. gluten or pollen). This can lead to autoimmunity and promote more inflammation in the body.

The problem is that you can't see this happening from the outside, but you can be sure it's happening on the inside and causing you to age faster (inflamm-age!).

And again, it's harder for women post menopause to control inflammation. Oestrogen is known to have anti-inflammatory effects, and studies have found that the decline in oestrogen levels after menopause can lead to an increase in inflammatory markers in the body.

The good news is that your diet and lifestyle can make a huge difference. Don't worry, we are going to cover that in Part 3.

Metabolic syndrome

Metabolic syndrome is a cluster of interconnected risk factors that significantly increase the likelihood of developing serious health conditions such as heart disease, stroke and type 2 diabetes.

These risk factors include obesity (especially around the middle), high blood pressure, high blood sugar levels, low HDL (good) cholesterol and elevated triglycerides. When a person has at least three of these factors, they are diagnosed with metabolic syndrome. These risk factors on their own are not good but having three together is a danger we need to avoid.

Unfortunately, it's very common. The NHS estimates that 1 in 3 adults over 50 has metabolic syndrome in the UK. The good news is that it's preventable. More on that in Part 3.

Muscle loss

One change that often goes overlooked as a key part of ageing is the loss of muscle mass and strength, which can have a significant impact on our overall health and wellbeing.

For women over 50, this is especially important. As we age, our bodies naturally begin to lose muscle mass, a condition known as sarcopenia. In fact, after the age of 30, you lose muscle mass at the rate of 3–8% per decade and this rate of decline is even higher after the age of 60.

As well as making it harder to do ordinary things, such as carrying things or climbing stairs, muscle loss has been linked to all kinds of health issues from cognitive decline and inflammation to immune issues.

But here's the good news: you don't have to accept muscle loss as an inevitable part of ageing.

In Part 3, we'll be looking at how you can incorporate weight training into your exercise routine, to help maintain your muscle mass and function well into your golden years.

Poor gut health

Over 1,500 years ago, Hippocrates said that "all diseases begin in the gut". Well, it turns out he was probably right! Our gut health plays a crucial role in our overall health, and a healthy gut microbiome is key to living a long and healthy life.

Poor gut health can have a big impact on how we age. It can

lead to chronic inflammation, which as we've seen raises the risk of age-related diseases like heart problems, Alzheimer's, and certain cancers. Plus, it can mess with our nutrient absorption, potentially causing deficiencies that affect our overall health.

But that's not all – a struggling gut can weaken our immune system, making it less effective at fighting off infections and more prone to triggering autoimmune issues. It can even mess with our brain, affecting our mental health, memory and risk of conditions like Alzheimer's. And when it comes to metabolism, our gut plays a role too, influencing our weight and the chance of developing things like diabetes.

Again, menopause can cause or aggravate gut issues. Oestrogen helps maintain the delicate balance of the microbiome and reduce inflammation, while progesterone helps to promote lactobacillus bacteria which helps to protect against low mood and anxiety. So declining hormones can upset the microbiome, interfere with brain health and promote more inflammation.

This all means that maintaining a healthy gut is a vital part of your healthy ageing toolkit.

Brain ageing

One of the most obvious things you might be noticing as you get older (and a key symptom of menopause) is the way your brain works (or doesn't!). Brain fog, memory loss, trouble concentrating, lack of focus; connections between neurons aren't quite firing as they used to.

And it can be scary. Especially if you have dementia in the family.

Certain forms of dementia do have a strong genetic component. Early-onset Alzheimer's for instance, which typically appears before the age of 65, is strongly influenced by genetics. However, early-onset Alzheimer's is relatively rare, accounting for less than 5% of all cases.

Late-onset Alzheimer's, which is the most common form of the disease, has a more complex genetic component. The presence of a particular variant of the APOE gene, known as the APOE ε4 allele, is associated with an increased risk of developing late-onset Alzheimer's disease. However, it's important to note that having the APOE ε4 allele far from guarantees that someone will develop Alzheimer's, and conversely, individuals without this variant can still develop the disease. The APOE ε4 allele is considered a risk factor rather than a definitive predictor.

However, while genetics can play a role in determining your risk of developing some forms of dementia as you age, it is definitely not the sole determining factor. There's a huge amount you can do to help those genes stay switched off (remember what I said about epigenetics?).

Let's have a look at what's happening to your brain as you age:

- **Oxidation.** Your brain cells are dying every day through oxidation (see the previous section on oxidation). Smoking, pollution, excess sugar, nutrient deficiencies and low levels of antioxidants can speed up oxidation, so there's plenty we can do to slow it down.
- **Inflammation.** Your brain is vulnerable to 'inflamm-aging' as much as the rest of your body. Depression, Alzheimer's and cognitive decline are all linked to chronic low-grade inflammation. Pro-inflammatory cytokines slow down your brain signalling and function, which can result in mood issues, forgetfulness, foggy thinking and anxiety. Adopting an anti-inflammatory diet and lifestyle is key to keeping inflammation at bay.
- **Sex hormone decline.** We will cover this in the hormone section, but the effects of lower levels of sex hormones on your brain can't be underestimated. Studies suggest that oestrogen, progesterone and testosterone play crucial roles in protecting women's brains against memory loss, cognitive decline and dementia.
- **Nutrient deficiencies.** As we get older, we may not be eating enough nutritious foods, and our ability to absorb nutrients also diminishes. This can deprive the brain of

essential nutrients such as omega-3 fats containing EPA and DHA, and vitamin D, both of which are essential for brain health.

- **Stress and your brain.** There's no getting away from it. Stress not only ages you, it also makes you foggy, forgetful and super grumpy! It also stops your brain cells working so you're more likely to get caught in negative thought patterns, impacting your focus, outlook, problem-solving, creativity and productivity. It also increases your risk of dementia and Alzheimer's disease.

Here's what excess cortisol tends to do to your brain:

- **Increases glutamate**, which can contribute to excitotoxicity and potentially lead to oxidation and neuronal damage.
- **Alters electrical signalling** that reduces memory and increases emotions.
- **Decreases BDNF** (brain-derived neurotrophic factor), a protein that's integral in keeping existing brain cells healthy and stimulating new brain cell formation.
- **Reduces serotonin and dopamine**, which can leave you depressed, unfocused, unmotivated and more prone to addictive behaviours.
- **Inhibits neurons** in the hippocampus, the part of your brain that stores memories.
- **Shrinks the prefrontal cortex,** which can negatively affect decision making, memory and control of impulsive behaviour.
- **Promotes leaky blood-brain barrier**. Just like your gut lining, the blood-brain barrier acts as your brain's gatekeeper, protecting your brain from harmful substances while letting needed nutrients in. Stress makes the blood-brain barrier more permeable, in effect making it leaky, increasing the risk of Alzheimer's disease, Parkinson's disease, multiple sclerosis and stroke.
- **Kills cells and shortens telomeres**. Stress can lead to premature ageing on a cellular level, increasing cell death and shortening telomere length.

Stress literally kills our brain cells and makes us more prone to cognitive decline and disease. Scary stuff. But it's why stress management is SO key to healthy ageing. And why I keep banging on about self-care and rest being non-negotiable …

While we might not expect our brain to work quite as it did in our 20s, we can definitely support our brain health with some diet, lifestyle and supplement tweaks (we'll cover this in Part 3).

Hormones – your Feisty Four

As we head into postmenopause, our hormones enter a new phase. The ebb and flow of our monthly cycle makes way for more settled, calmer waters. It's like we've reached the end of the turbulent rapids and are now floating gently towards the calm sea, sipping a cocktail and enjoying the view.

Unfortunately, hormones are still running the show in the background, determining how calm that sea is and how lovely the view!

I wrote in detail about hormones in my first book, highlighting four hormones that stand out as the main drivers for how we look, feel, think and behave. I named them the Feisty Four, and they are just as important now you're through the turbulence of your monthly cycle.

Your Feisty Four play a crucial role in the ageing process, influencing cellular ageing, inflammation and metabolism, as well as bone health, muscle mass and cognitive function.

Here's a quick reminder of what they are and how they can affect you now you're postmenopausal (read more about them in my book, *It's Not You, It's Your Hormones*, or skip this section if you've already read the book).

Cortisol

If you've been in my community at all, you'll know I talk about this hormone almost every time I touch on women's health – and for a reason. It's THE dominant hormone and will run riot over all your other hormones if you don't keep it under control. When cortisol is out of balance, it can cause multiple symptoms pretty much anywhere, from anxiety, mood swings and brain fog to hair loss and IBS.

Cortisol is your main stress hormone. It's your survival hormone, your body's primary tool in dealing with any stress or threat. It's part of your evolutionary fight-or-flight response to danger, and it's vital to keep you alive.

In caveman times, it saved your life when you were attacked by a lion or had to endure long bouts of famine.

These days, not so many lion attacks (or famines), but cortisol instead keeps you going when you have a million modern day micro stresses to deal with. From your alarm going off in the morning, to traffic jams, work deadlines, arguments with loved ones, and the multitude of tasks we need to get through as part of the daily juggle.

Our bodies have evolved and adapted in many ways since caveman times, but our adrenal stress response is exactly the same. The brain can't distinguish between a lion attack and an argument with your loved one.

The real problem is that we don't get any 'cave' time to switch off. A holiday once in a while is great, but it's not enough to properly rebalance your stress response. Unless you're scheduling regular daily relaxation, you are probably running non-stop on adrenaline and cortisol.

Cortisol is good in the right amounts. We need it to wake up in the morning and keep us alert and energised until bedtime. It's unrelenting high levels of cortisol over a prolonged period that can have negative effects on our health. Not only is it exhausting for your body, but it accelerates the ageing process.

Stress hormones carry the message to your DNA and your cells that your body is under attack. This message directly affects how your genes express proteins and how your cells function. In survival mode, every cell in your body is on alert and is directing energy and resources to your emergency functions, i.e. your fight-or-flight response. There is very little left for rest, regeneration, repair and maintenance of your body systems such as digestion, immunity, brain function and detoxification processes.

Therefore, as well as switching on genes that promote disease and accelerate ageing, here's what excess cortisol is doing to your body:

- **Skin ageing:** Too much cortisol can make your skin lose its elasticity and become more prone to wrinkles.
- **Brain health:** We've already seen how cortisol actually damages brain neurons and reduces your ability to think clearly and efficiently.
- **Heart health:** Chronic stress and high cortisol levels have been linked to an increased risk of hypertension, heart disease and stroke.
- **Weight:** Not only do we tend to eat more (and less healthily) when we're stressed, cortisol also likes to store fat around the belly area, which is a risk factor for diabetes and heart disease.
- **Bone health:** High levels of cortisol can increase the breakdown of bone tissue and decrease bone density, both risk factors for fractures and osteoporosis.
- **Immune system:** Too much cortisol for too long can increase inflammation and weaken your immune response, making it harder for you to fight off illness and disease. In fact, it's SO effective at doing this that doctors use stress hormones (e.g. steroids) in organ transplants to stop the immune system attacking the new organ. It's also used to reduce inflammation in conditions like eczema and arthritis.
- **Digestive system:** Cortisol can mess with your digestion and cause problems like acid reflux, ulcers and irritable

bowel syndrome (IBS).

- **Sex hormones:** After menopause, when your ovaries stop producing oestrogen and progesterone, the adrenal glands become the primary source of oestrogen and progesterone. If your adrenal glands are already overtaxed, it can severely impact this back-up source of sex hormone production and prolong menopause symptoms.

What's stressing you out?
Sources of stress for women over 40 can include;.

1. Physical stressors:
- Menopause
- Ageing
- Health conditions
- Infections or illness
- Injuries and surgeries
- Pregnancy and childbirth
- Environmental, including toxins, chemicals, mould, allergies
- Nutritional – poor diet, nutrient deficiencies, food intolerances, blood sugar imbalance, dehydration, alcohol
- Digestive stress – microbiome imbalance, inflammation
- Medications

2. Emotional stressors:
- Family and relationships
- Grief or bereavement
- Financial worries
- Work stress
- Technology, including social media
- Emotions such as feeling lonely, worried, angry, frustrated, unfulfilled, rejected, sad, bored, insecure, guilty, fearful, unloved or carrying around unresolved emotional or psychological stress such as past trauma or PTSD.

Knowing your sources of stress can help you minimise or manage them. Then finding effective coping mechanisms and prioritising a small amount of time to rest and relaxation each day, can make a significant difference in managing cortisol and helping you age healthily.

I'll be covering some of the most common emotional stressors in the next section.

Thyroid

Think of your thyroid hormones as the regulators of your body's engine. When there's plenty of them, they rev up your engine, leading to a higher metabolism, increased energy, enhanced alertness and a warmer body temperature.

Conversely, when thyroid hormones are low, they are in conservation mode, slowing down your engine, conserving energy, reducing temperature and shutting down non-essential functions.

These hormones essentially determine whether your body's engine runs at full throttle or conserves fuel as you age, making them pivotal in the ageing process.

Hypothyroidism is a lot more common than *hyperthyroidism.* Hypothyroidism is when you have an underactive thyroid or low output of thyroid hormones (T4 and T3). Hyperthyroidism is when you've got too much thyroid hormone, causing potential symptoms such as anxiety, palpitations, sweating, weight loss or hyperactivity.

Women are more at risk of thyroid conditions than men, but are particularly prone to hypothyroidism, especially as we age or if it runs in the family.

As thyroid hormones travel to every cell in the body, hypothyroidism can have a wide range of symptoms. The most common ones are:

- fatigue
- weight gain
- brain fog
- memory loss
- depression
- hair loss
- cold hands/feet
- dry skin
- brittle nails
- PMS
- anxiety
- mood swings
- puffy face or skin
- missing outer third of eyebrow
- aching joints
- low sex drive
- constipation
- high cholesterol

As we age, our thyroid hormone pathway gets less efficient and is further affected by other stuff going on in the body such as illness, diet, stress, digestive health, organ reserve, toxins and menopause.

Unfortunately, this isn't a one-way street. If thyroid function declines, it can accelerate the ageing process itself. Left untreated, hypothyroidism not only brings about unpleasant symptoms, it can also raise the risk of more serious conditions such as obesity, heart disease, osteoporosis, dementia and diabetes.

It's therefore important to get your thyroid properly tested if you have symptoms. Jump to Part 3 Balance for more on supporting your thyroid, and the Going Deeper chapter for more on testing.

Insulin

Insulin is a hormone dispatched by your pancreas whenever you eat foods made up of carbohydrates and protein. Its job is to pick up glucose and amino acids from the blood and deliver them to your liver and muscle cells. Cells take what they require for energy conversion, while any surplus is stashed away in your fat cells for future needs.

The problem is that when you're taking in too much sugar or refined carbohydrates, or enduring prolonged periods of stress (which also puts sugar in your blood), your body might end up with an overabundance of insulin coursing through your system.

There are four main problems that excess insulin can cause:

1. Weight gain/obesity: If you already have enough energy stores in your cells (from your last meal or snack), insulin will need to store it in your fat cells (making them bigger!).

2. Blood sugar imbalance/risk of diabetes: Too much sugar or carbs in your diet can result in a blood sugar roller coaster, with too much insulin being produced. This can increase your risk of type 2 diabetes, obesity, heart disease, cancer and dementia.

3. Inflammation: Insulin can promote more inflammation, which we know can contribute to faster ageing and chronic disease. As well as bad news for your heart, inflammation can impact your brain – especially cognitive function like memory.

4. Insulin resistance and metabolic syndrome: A major risk factor for obesity, diabetes, heart disease, dementia and cancer.

As we go through menopause, we are more prone to insulin resistance. This is when your cells become less sensitive or receptive to insulin. They can't keep up with all the carbs and sugar coming along. The insulin receptors on your cells shut down, and that leads to more insulin production to try to deal with the extra unwanted sugar.

This is exacerbated by common ageing factors such as a slower metabolism, increased fat to muscle ratio, or being less active or more stressed. We just can't handle carbs like we used to!

Insulin resistance can be referred to as pre-diabetes or hyperinsulinemia. It's also a key component in metabolic syndrome, and has been directly linked to the onset of Alzheimer's disease (sometimes unofficially referred to by researchers as type 3 diabetes).

These are some of the symptoms or signs relating to an insulin or blood sugar imbalance:

- High waist:hip ratio (although you don't need to be overweight to have insulin resistance)
- High blood pressure
- High cholesterol or triglycerides
- Elevated HbA1c
- Feeling tired, 'hangry' or dizzy if you don't eat
- Excessive thirst and/or frequent urination
- Constant sugar or carb cravings
- Family history of type 2 diabetes or hyperinsulinemia

Unfortunately, if you have lots of sugar in your blood, it can accelerate ageing via a process called 'glycation' or as I like to call it, 'death by sugar'! This is when glucose molecules can attach themselves to proteins and cause damage or stop them working at all (remember those faulty clumping proteins we covered in Part 1?). The end result is the production of AGE (Advanced Glycation End) products, and the more they accumulate, the faster we age.

In Part 3, we'll look at how to balance your blood sugar to help you to manage your insulin and avoid glycation and other issues.

Sex hormones

Our sex hormones are at their optimum during our reproductive phase, so it's logical that once they decline post menopause, we are going to be more at risk of accelerated ageing.

Here's how declining sex hormones can impact how you age:

Oestrogen

Oestrogen is our 'youth hormone'. As well as having a key role in your monthly cycle (preparing you for reproducing), it helps your skin feel plump and smooth, your hair feels thick and shiny, your bones and joints strong and resilient, and your heart healthy. On top of that it has a vital role in your mood, brain function and sex drive, as well as protecting your immune system.

When we get to midlife and start producing less oestrogen, we can really start feeling the effects: increased wrinkles, sagging or dry skin, thinning hair, mood swings, anxiety, memory loss, brain fog, joint pain, vaginal dryness and low libido. It can feel like we're ageing overnight!

Not only can we start to feel older, but declining sex hormone levels can lead to chronic inflammation, shortened telomeres and metabolic disruptions, increasing the risk of age-related diseases like heart disease, cancer and metabolic disorders.

Progesterone

As we progress through menopause, progesterone levels decline rapidly, since its production is tied to ovulation. Once we stop ovulating, we can produce small amounts in other parts of the body, however levels are likely to be low.

Progesterone is often considered nature's antidepressant, as it enhances mood and reduces anxiety. It also promotes the calming hormone GABA, which helps reduce stress and induce sleep. Declining levels can result in symptoms such as anxiety, poor sleep as well as other health issues.

Progesterone has been shown to have vasodilatory effects, meaning it can relax blood vessels, potentially leading to lower blood pressure and better heart health. It's also anti-inflammatory and protects your bones, working with oestrogen to maintain a balance between bone resorption and formation.

Testosterone
Testosterone is not just a male hormone! Yes, it's mainly associated with male characteristics such as facial hair, a deep voice, sperm production, libido and the maintenance of muscle mass and strength. However, it plays a crucial role for women too, including bone and brain health as well as sex drive, mood, sleep and energy. We only make about 5% of the levels men make, but it's a hormone that we definitely need. And just like oestrogen and progesterone, testosterone levels decline during and post menopause, and this can result in a variety of health issues and symptoms.

Supporting healthy sex hormone levels is important for all women. Your genes, diet and lifestyle can play a big part here, as can medical support such as HRT.

We will be addressing how to support many of these ageing factors in the EMBRACE protocol in Part 3.

PSYCHOLOGICAL AGEING

As the years pass, physical changes will occur to varying degrees, influenced by your genetics, diet, lifestyle and environment. However, as we've seen, one of the most significant factors in how well you age is stress – and how you manage it. The wear and tear that stress places on your body and mind can not only affect how old you feel, but also determine your susceptibility to chronic diseases.

One of the best analogies I've heard likens constant stress to your body being in a state of perpetual warfare. All the troops are busy fighting on the front line, consuming a huge amount of energy. There are very few resources left for the long-term projects like repair and rebuilding, much needed to protect against the damage and risks that come with ageing.

And the battle never ceases; it's a perpetual struggle. As you soldier on, your body gradually weakens with time.

But where is all this stress coming from? Unlike our ancestors, whose main source of stress was physical – either being killed by a predator, infection or famine – modern-day stress is mainly emotional.

Whether they arise from your past, trauma or your current circumstances, emotional or psychological stressors are just as powerful as physical stressors such as injury or infection. They trigger the same physical stress response – your fight-or-flight response kicks in and you produce stress hormones.

And let's face it, there's no shortage of emotional stressors in midlife for a woman! By the time you've reached middle age, it's probable that you've encountered various forms of trauma or loss, such as the death of a loved one, significant life changes, divorce, abuse, discrimination, fertility or family challenges, empty nest syndrome, financial struggles and more, which will undoubtedly impact your thoughts and emotions.

You may be unhappy about how your body is changing, or you may be experiencing feelings of loneliness, invisibility or irrelevance as an older woman. On top of that, you may have more responsibilities at work or be stuck in the sandwich of caring for kids and elderly parents.

Whatever stresses you face in your life, what's important is how you perceive and respond to them. This ultimately determines their impact on your health and wellbeing.

The mind-body connection

We have known for many years that the mind has a powerful influence on the body. You only have to look at the placebo effect to see how this works. Many studies have shown how patient beliefs and expectations can produce real changes in health outcomes, even when the treatment itself has no direct therapeutic properties.

One study involved patients with migraines. For each of six migraine attacks, they were given either a powerful painkiller, a placebo or no treatment. Various labels were attributed to the pills to assess whether this made a difference. Results showed that the real painkiller was the most effective, however when it was labelled as 'placebo', it provided the same amount of relief as the placebo labelled as the drug. The belief in the label was just as strong as the drug itself.

A review of eight studies on antidepressant treatment revealed that over a 12-week period, placebo treatments were just as effective in relieving depression symptoms. Another review of cough medication trials revealed that 85% of cough reduction was attributed to the placebo effect, while only 15% was due to the active ingredient.

Psychoneuroimmunology (PNI) explores the complex inter-actions between the nervous system, the endocrine system and the immune system, and how these interactions are influenced by our thoughts and emotions. It bridges the gap between psychology and physiology, providing insights into how mental states can have tangible effects on physical health.

Bruce H. Lipton's *The Biology of Belief* is a fascinating look at how our physical health is affected by our mind. He challenges conventional scientific wisdom, arguing that cells are influenced not solely by DNA but also by external factors, including thoughts and beliefs. He emphasises the power that positive thinking can have on our biology and overall health, and recommends practices such as mindfulness, positive thinking, stress management and activities that help us process our emotions such as counselling, therapy and journaling.

Another one of my favourites is Dr Gabor Maté's book, *When the Body Says No: Understanding the Stress-Disease Connection.*

Gabor Maté, a respected physician and author, brings to light the critical link between chronic emotional stress, trauma and the development of physical illnesses. He points out that the roots of many health issues, including autoimmune diseases, cancer and heart conditions, can often be traced back to emotional stress, particularly from early life experiences and/or trauma.

In the book I was particularly struck by the story of Mary, who developed scleroderma, an autoimmune disease that causes stiffening of the skin, oesophagus, heart, lungs and other tissues. Maté describes how Mary, a dedicated nurse, had been abused as a child, and had to protect her sisters from the same fate. She consistently put the needs of others before her own and suppressed her emotions, particularly anger and resentment, to maintain harmony in her personal and professional life.

Maté uses Mary's story to demonstrate how chronic emotional suppression can contribute to physical disease. He explains that the continual stress of repressing emotions, especially negative ones like anger, can have a profound impact on the immune system, potentially leading to autoimmune diseases like the one Mary experienced.

Deepak Chopra, in *Ageless Body, Timeless Mind*, writes about the concept of 'quantum healing', proposing that the mind has a profound influence on the body's ageing process. He explores how thoughts, emotions and beliefs can affect gene expression, hormonal balance and cellular function, ultimately shaping the ageing trajectory. He illustrates how practices such as meditation, mindfulness and conscious living can promote physical rejuvenation, mental clarity and emotional wellbeing.

Marisa Peer, in her book *You Can Be Younger*, explains that how we psychologically age determines how we physically age. Our thoughts become feelings, and feelings affect our biochemistry. The mind believes what you tell it, and then tells your body to reflect those thoughts. So, the beliefs and thoughts we have about ageing can make us age faster or slower, depending on whether they are positive or negative. If our thoughts are fearful or negative (for example, if you tell yourself you look old in the mirror) or your belief is that you are too old to do something, your body will act accordingly. We can literally think ourselves older.

We can conclude from these authors and scientific research that what you think and how you feel have a powerful impact on your health. Your thoughts are a form of energy, and each one produces a chemical reaction in your body, which in turn influences how your genes are expressed (epigenetics).

Positive feelings such as love, joy, connection, gratitude and fulfilment trigger feel good hormones such as serotonin, dopamine, oxytocin and growth hormone. These hormones not only make you feel good, but they can alter your gene expression to promote resilience and health.

Conversely, negative feelings such as fear, anger, sadness, grief, loneliness, guilt, inadequacy, frustration, low self-esteem, rejection, guilt, worry, self-doubt and heartbreak will trigger your stress hormones cortisol, adrenalin and noradrenalin. And with them come a host of inflammatory cytokines that keep you in the fight-or-flight loop, and switch on genes that can promote disease.

And it's a vicious or virtuous cycle depending on the nature of your thoughts.

Let's break that down. Say you have a simple thought like 'I'm looking ugly/old/fat today', that triggers a feeling in your body of sadness or low self-esteem, which signals your brain to release stress hormones which travel to your cells and switch on genes that create imbalance (inflammation, etc.). The emotion of sadness or low self-worth then creates more thoughts about how ugly/old/fat you look, and the vicious cycle begins. And this can go on for years, with every new thought reinforcing the emotion until it becomes an automatic programme (or limiting belief), running from your subconscious. And now we're more at risk of imbalance and disease.

And this is just one train of thought. We might have hundreds of negative thoughts every day, relating to how we see ourselves, what's on our social media feed, the news, how we interact with our partner, family, boss, colleagues, worries about money, health, relationships or work stresses – the list goes on. Imagine all those negative loops running every single day!

The good news is that the reverse is also true. If we think happy thoughts, like 'I look good today' or 'I love my life' or simply being grateful for something, it creates feelings of love, gratitude, joy, which then tells your brain to release happy hormones like serotonin, dopamine and oxytocin. These hormones can switch on genes that promote health and balance. And now we have a 'virtuous' cycle where we not only feel happy but we are literally creating health in our bodies. The mind is totally connected to and in sync with the body in a positive way.

In addition to that, according to the book *The Telomere Effect* by scientists Elizabeth Blackburn and Elissa Epel, negative thoughts can shorten your telomeres! Having a pessimistic outlook, nurturing cynical thoughts, constantly worrying, suppressing your emotions, and failing to live in the moment are all factors that can potentially shorten your telomeres, and consequently, your lifespan.

Negative emotions are simply part of being human – we all feel them from time to time, especially as we get older and have more life experiences. It's when they are prolonged or remain unresolved that they can start to take a toll on our health.

But, if we can transform negative thoughts into positive ones, then we can not only feel better today, but increase our chances of a long and healthy life in the future.

Much more on that in Part 3.

In the meantime, let's have a closer look at some of the emotions that may be prominent for you at this time in your life.

Self-doubt

Research suggests that women are more likely to experience heightened self-doubt during midlife compared to other life stages. This is no doubt due to a mix of societal expectations, hormonal changes, life transitions, limiting beliefs, low self-worth and ageism.

Self-doubt, poor self-esteem and low confidence will not only create more stress in your body but can also stop you achieving your goals and feeling fulfilled. They are limiting beliefs that can sabotage your happiness and your health.

It's inherently human to experience these limiting beliefs, we all have voices in our head that tell us we're not good enough, not capable, not lovable, not worthy, don't fit in, etc. They may come from our childhood, or past experiences, and they can stay with us forever, dictating our choices and how we feel, live and behave. They exist as part of our protection system, to stop us experiencing negative emotions, but they can end up stopping us living a fully happy and fulfilled life.

Tara Mohr talks about these voices as 'inner critics' in her excellent book *Playing Big:* "The inner critic is cunning. If it simply said to you, 'No, don't compose the song, don't run for office, don't make the career change, don't share your ideas – it's too risky,' you wouldn't listen. You'd probably reply with something along the lines of, 'No, I feel okay about the risks. Here I go.' So, the safety instinct uses a more effective argument: 'Your paintings are terrible.' 'Your book won't offer anything new – there are so many books on the subject.' 'Your attempt at a career change will cause you to end up broke.' The inner critic speaks up with more viciousness and volume when we are exposing ourselves to a real or perceived vulnerability – something that triggers a fear of embarrassment, rejection, failure or pain."

Tony Robbins, author and coach, says of self-doubt: "Self-doubt is learned. No one is born with self-doubt – children typically move through the world with plenty of confidence.

By the time we reach adulthood, our natural confidence has been undermined by the opinions of others and by our own experiences … Wherever it comes from, self-doubt is a defence mechanism. It's our brains protecting us – from failure, from embarrassment, from heartbreak. But it's also driven by fear, and it prevents us from achieving excellence."

'Not good enough' is a common inner critic for many women. It tends to result in self-doubt and people-pleasing, influenced by societal norms and gender expectations. From a young age, girls may learn to prioritise others' needs over their own, seeking external validation to counter feelings of inadequacy. This can lead to a cycle of people-pleasing behaviours where women suppress their own desires in order to gain approval and maintain harmony, which in turn reinforces feelings of self-doubt.

The good news is there are lots of ways that you can break this cycle and overcome self-doubt and other limiting beliefs. In Part 3, we'll look at cultivating self-awareness, changing your thoughts and self-talk, setting boundaries, creating more joy in your life, seeking out supportive networks and deeper connections, and building your resilience.

Loneliness

Loneliness in modern society is not just about being alone. It's not something you can measure by counting how many friends you've got or how many likes you get on Instagram. If you feel lonely, then you're lonely, plain and simple. Even if you're surrounded by people or in a loving relationship, you can still feel lonely, disconnected from others (or yourself), misunderstood, neglected, not heard or seen by those around you.

We all experience loneliness from time to time, but it's when those feelings stick around for the long haul that it starts to have an impact on our mental and physical health.

This can be attributed to our evolutionary history, where being disconnected from the group posed a significant threat to our survival. In those times, belonging was as crucial as having food to eat. So, when we feel isolated, we enter a state that historically signified grave danger, activating our stress mechanisms.

And there's evidence to support this. Several studies have found that social isolation and loneliness are linked to a higher risk of mortality, especially in middle-aged and older adults. In fact, one study showed that people who reported feeling lonely or isolated had a 26% increased risk of dying over a six-year period.

Another study in the *European Heart Journal* on patients with type 2 diabetes concluded that "loneliness is worse for your heart than lack of exercise".

Feelings of belonging are being eroded as friendship groups are shrinking, and it's particularly worse if you're in midlife and live in the UK. The UK government's 2021 Friendship Study reported that 1 in 8 Britons said they had only one close friend, while 7% had no friends at all. A 2023 study by Arizona State University found that midlifers in England (45-to-65-year-olds) are the loneliest in Europe, more so than any other generation.

We don't seem to have quite recovered from the aftermath of the Covid pandemic, which hugely exacerbated social isolation. Where we used to meet up for shopping trips, or exercise classes, many of us are still opting for the convenience or comfort of doing this online.

Psychologist Marisa G Franco, author of the book Platonic, believes that "loneliness makes us withdraw and perceive other people as threatening. We devalue how important connection is, we choose not to depend on other people, which makes us lonelier. It's a vicious cycle."

In Okinawa, Japan, one of the five Blue Zone regions known for longevity, they recognise that loneliness is a particular problem for ageing adults. They even have a word for it, *kodokushi*, which means lonely deaths among older people. They combat this by creating *moais*, unique support groups that can stay together for a lifetime.

Staying socially connected and avoiding loneliness and isolation are key steps to a longer, happier life (we'll cover this in the Connect part of the EMBRACE protocol in Part 3).

Trauma

If you've experienced trauma or chronic stress in your life, you have a higher risk of developing mental health conditions such as post-traumatic stress disorder (PTSD), depression, anxiety disorders, and other mood disorders, all of which can accelerate the ageing process.

The good news is that the more coping methods you have to improve your resilience, such as social support, cognitive flexibility and adaptive coping strategies, the more you can mitigate the negative impacts of trauma and stress as you age.

If you have or are suffering trauma-related stress, it's important to seek professional help (I've included some links in the Resources section at the end of the book).

Family and relationships

There's no denying that a big source of emotional stress can often be related to family, relationships and children if you have them.

Whether you grew up in a loving or challenging environment, family dynamics play a significant role in shaping your emotional wellbeing, bringing either joy or stress into your life (and often both!).

Not surprisingly, when friends and family are a source of negativity in your life, you're more at risk of being unhealthy. When they are a source of support and encouragement, the reverse is true.

For those who've chosen to have children later in life, young ones can be physically demanding. The struggle to balance work, family and dwindling energy reserves can be compounded if you lack support or are navigating the menopause.

On the other hand, if you've had children earlier, you may find yourself going through perimenopause when your children become teenagers. This can be a big hormonal clash!

For those who've faced infertility, it can also be an emotional roller coaster. Feelings of loss and isolation can run deep, but seeking support can help to provide relief.

Relationship endings, divorce and heartbreak can have a significant impact on the stress levels and ageing process for women (at any age!). The emotional turmoil, grief and feelings of loss, betrayal or anger can take a huge toll on a woman's wellbeing, both mentally and physically.

When (and if) the kids finally leave home, it can be a bittersweet moment for many women. On the one hand, there's a sense of pride and accomplishment in seeing your children embark on their own journey. But on the other hand, there's an overwhelming mix of emotions that can hit hard, often referred to as the 'empty nest syndrome'. It can feel like a big void, leaving a sense of loss and loneliness, along with uncertainty about your future purpose or identity.

It's a time of transition that often coincides with the physical changes that are happening in menopause. And this can be especially challenging. While some women embrace their newfound freedom, others might struggle with who they are now that their primary role as a caregiver has shifted. It's important to acknowledge and validate these feelings, seeking support from loved ones, friends or professional counsellors who can provide guidance and help to navigate this new chapter.

This is a good time for you to discover new passions, reconnect with neglected hobbies and find a renewed sense of self.

The empty nest might be daunting at first, but it's also a huge opportunity for personal growth and self-discovery. Time to focus on you!

Whatever your situation, it's important to recognise your emotions and get the help or support you need to deal with them so you can have a happier and more positive future. As we have seen, it's our response to these stresses, via our thoughts and emotions, that is the key to how they affect us. If we can be happier from the inside out, we can reduce our reliance on other people or external circumstances to make us feel good.

We'll look at some strategies you can adopt in the Rest and Connect pieces of the EMBRACE protocol in Part 3.

Grief

We've all heard those stories about older people who seem to 'die of a broken heart' when they lose a loved one. In science, this is referred to as 'broken heart syndrome' or 'takotsubo cardiomyopathy'.

While bereavement is a commonly recognised form of grief, there are various other types of grief that women can experience. These could include divorce/end of relationships, family feuds, loss of health, stillbirth or miscarriage, loss of friendship, moving house or being displaced, change in financial status, loss of job, empty nest, retirement or infertility.

Working on your emotional health and resilience can really help you to cope with these feelings and there are many grief and bereavement support resources that can help you if you're struggling. Skip to Resources for more info.

Work stress

Menopausal women are the fastest growing workforce demographic. With state pension age constantly being pushed back and retirement savings often falling short, this will only continue as many of us will face a much longer working life.

And we are feeling the stress. By the time you reach midlife, as well as dealing with menopause symptoms, you may be in a role with higher levels of responsibility after many years of working hard to progress your career, often juggling home and family responsibilities on top of work stresses. Or you may have had to leave or change your job due to your health issues.

This was reflected in the Health and Safety Executive report in 2015 that found that midlife women reported more work-related stress than any other group.

This isn't a surprise. Not only are women's brains more susceptible to negative stimuli, but as Tamu Thomas in her excellent book *Women Who Work Too Much* states, women "live in a society that conditions us from early childhood to value productivity above all else, to temper our emotions, to not be 'needy', and to think rest is simply to recharge our batteries so that we can get back to commodifying ourselves for profit we will not enjoy."

While we must encourage organisations to offer women more support, it's crucial to take responsibility for your own wellbeing. Even if you're fortunate enough to work in a supportive company, it's still up to you to make the most of the resources available. And if you're stuck in a less-than-ideal work situation, remember, you still have the power to make changes. Progress might not be quick or easy, but there are always options available to you, both for your health and for your overall life journey.

The culture of busy

In today's culture, particularly for women, there's a subtle, yet powerful, glorification of being perpetually busy. We often wear 'busy' as a badge of honour, without which we might feel useless or unimportant. Our lives can be an endless cycle of busyness, addicted to the adrenaline rush it brings. This compulsion to always be 'on' or active can make moments of rest or relaxation feel dull or laden with guilt. Or worse, it can make us feel like a failure.

There is a deep-rooted mix of social conditioning, cultural expectations and traditional gender roles at play here. Our 'people-pleasing' mentality can make it challenging for us to focus on our own needs without feeling selfish. Cultural norms reinforce this by idealising women as selfless caregivers and nurturers, making it difficult to step away from these roles without feeling guilty or facing resistance or judgement.

On top of this, we are constantly told we can 'have it all'. To have a great career, family, health and social life is the ultimate marker of success. But to do that we have to be superwomen! And this constant pressure to succeed in each area can be more draining than empowering. We can often end up not doing anything very well. And then feeling guilty about all of it.

The truth is, in our pursuit to do it all while pleasing everybody, we miss out on downtime. When we're addicted to being busy, it's hard to appreciate or engage in slower, quieter moments. But constantly chasing this adrenaline high is a fast track to burnout and increased risk of chronic disease.

Lorraine Candy, author of *What's Wrong With Me? 101 Things Midlife Women Need To Know,* says: "I still can't find a woman who has quietly given herself the permission to relax, without guilt, without apology or without having to explain to the world that she has earned the right to prioritise pleasure, play, rest and selfish joy during moments of her daily life ... we continue to praise being busy, we hero the hectic, we attach our self-worth to productivity, but we don't celebrate calmness, quietness when we see it. We don't value 'liquid ease' (my fantasy of a relaxed woman) if we see it; this kind of personality trait is worth less."

Tamu Thomas talks about toxic productivity as "the unconscious, obsessive-compulsive desire to be productive *all the time.* It's when you build your life around work and forget the purpose of work is to make a living in order to live. It's the process of being detached from the present and focusing on the future. A future that holds the promise that 'one day' you'll have worked enough and achieved enough success to feel fulfilled and worthy enough to enjoy your life."

There's a deeper reason many of us are invested in being 'busy' all the time. It's a distraction from facing our feelings. When you're moving so fast, and constantly busy, you don't have the time or space to connect and deal with your feelings, or the emotions you're trying to avoid – whether that's sadness, anger, frustration, loneliness, guilt, poor self-worth or some other emotion that's uncomfortable for you. But the longer you repress these emotions, the more you're likely to risk damaging your physical health.

It's vital to understand that taking a break, slowing down, setting some healthy boundaries, isn't just okay – it's essential. Embracing rest and downtime, saying no to 'people-pleasing' without guilt is vital for our mental and physical health, especially as we get older. And if you need some professional help in order to face your emotions head on, then this is the time to get it.

We'll cover some strategies for this under Rest and Connect in the EMBRACE protocol in Part 3.

Technology
Technology has brought many positive changes to our lives, from making communication faster and more convenient to improving access to information. In a world where our smartphones and tablets have become constant companions, this digital closeness comes with a hidden cost to our mental and physical health.

According to the UK's communications regulator, Ofcom, the average person in the UK checks their phone every 12 minutes, often first thing in the morning and last thing at night.

There's even a new word, coined by YouGov researchers, to describe the anxiety felt when we don't have our phones –

'nomophobia' stands for 'no mobile phone phobia'!

We've just been talking about stress at work. Thanks to our smartphones and laptops, we're always within reach of our employers. Yes, it brings flexibility, but it also means we struggle to disconnect from work, keeping that fight-or-flight mode well and truly switched on.

Additionally, the constant stream of news and information can leave us feeling overwhelmed and exhausted. And we all know how stressful social media can be. While it keeps us connected, excessive use has been linked to feelings of anxiety, depression and loneliness. We see everyone's highlight reel, and it can make us feel like we're not measuring up or missing out. Seeing others do things we wish we were doing can hugely impact our self-esteem.

And all this is really messing with our sleep. Scrolling on our phones or using tablets before bedtime can screw up your sleep-wake cycle, and inhibit the production of melatonin, your sleep hormone.

Technology can also make us couch potatoes. With streaming services, online shopping, meal deliveries and more, we don't have to go anywhere these days! Plus, there are concerns about the huge increase in radiation exposure from mobile phones and devices. Some studies suggest it could increase our cancer risk.

And let's not overlook addiction. Checking your phone or emails can be totally addictive, pushing up your stress levels and instead of making you feel more connected, it's likely doing the opposite. This constant urge to check our phones is driven by brain chemistry. Specifically, dopamine, often referred to as the 'feel-good' molecule because of its role in the brain's reward system, plays a significant part in this behaviour. Dopamine is the same molecule that gets released when we take drugs and alcohol. However, the more 'digital dopamine' we get, the more we use up, and the more we crave, and our addiction grows.

There's more! Prolonged device use can affect our eyes, causing strain and fatigue. The noise pollution from all those notifications can stress us out. And our posture can suffer too, leading to all sorts of back, neck and shoulder pain.

But one of the worst impacts of technology in my view, is the way we can miss out on being present, both with others and the world around us. I see it with couples out at restaurants, on their own phones in their own worlds, not talking to each other. And this disconnection from the present moment can seriously impact our relationships, health and happiness.

We have to embrace the positives technology is bringing us, but we also have to be very aware of how it affects us and put measures in place to make sure we're OK. Let's come back to how we can manage this better in Part 3.

PART 2

HEALTH CHECK:

Where Are You Now?

CHAPTER 4:

TAKE THE QUIZ

Congratulations if you've made it through the turbulence of menopause! While some of the more challenging symptoms may have disappeared (no more period hell), unfortunately you may still be experiencing lingering issues or even new ones long after menopause.

In this section, we'll take a quick quiz to identify some of the most common body and mind issues you may be facing, and then look at some tools to get you feeling better. Now is the time to deal with anything you've been ignoring or haven't yet found solutions for. Symptoms are your body's way of telling you something isn't in balance. We need to start taking notice of them and getting back in control so we're in the best shape for the years ahead.

This questionnaire is not designed to diagnose you. It is just a tool to give you an indication of where you may have an imbalance and how you can help yourself using the tips provided (and the EMBRACE protocol in Part 3). I fully recommend you get personalised advice from a qualified medical or health practitioner if you have unresolved symptoms or have serious health conditions.

If you answer a, b or c to any of these questions, jump to the section in Chapter 5 on that symptom for more info on how to improve it.

How are your energy levels?

a/ I'm exhausted most of the time
b/ I'm tired often, and rely on coffee, sugar or naps to get through the day
c/ My energy levels are generally OK, but have occasional slumps during the day
d/ I have plenty of energy all day long

How do you sleep?

a/ I struggle to get more than six hours sleep a night
b/ I struggle to fall asleep and/or wake up several times during the night
c/ I fall asleep easily but occasionally wake up
d/ I sleep well most nights

How is your brain working?

a/ I feel foggy and forgetful most of the time
b/ I'm often forgetting things and have trouble focusing
c/ I occasionally have forgetful moments or lapses in concentration
d/ I'm sharp and focused, and have no problem remembering things

How happy are you with your weight?

a/ I'm overweight and really fed up with it
b/ My weight is creeping up and I'm not happy with it
c/ I am OK generally, but have a bit of belly fat that won't shift
d/ I'm happy with my weight

How is your mood?

a/ I suffer every day with mood swings, anger or bouts of depression
b/ I'm often irritable, snappy and/or emotional
c/ I occasionally feel irritable, low, flat or overemotional
d/ I feel happy and balanced most of the time

How are your stress/anxiety levels?

a/ I'm experiencing stress and/or anxiety on a daily basis
b/ I feel more stressed and anxious than I have in the past

c/ I occasionally feel overwhelmed and/or anxious

d/ I feel mostly calm and balanced, and deal with stress well

How are you down under?

a/ I regularly have a mix of genito-urinary symptoms (e.g. leakage, vulval issues, pain, irritation, itching, prolapse, bladder or urinary tract infections (UTIs))

b/ I am often caught out with one or more of these symptoms

c/ I have the occasional symptom

d/ I never suffer from these issues

How is your sex drive?

a/ I have no sex drive and/or have vaginal dryness/sex is painful

b/ I have low libido and/or some vaginal dryness

c/ My sex drive is OK but not where I'd like it to be

d/ I have a healthy sex drive and no vaginal dryness

How is your gut health?

a/ I have diagnosed digestive issues (e.g. IBS/IBD) and or severe food sensitivities/allergies

b/ I often have digestive issues or reactions to foods, but nothing diagnosed or treated

c/ I have occasional digestive issues or food sensitivities

d/ I have no digestive issues and can eat what I want

How are your joints and bones?

a/ I have severe chronic joint pain and/or osteoporosis

b/ I often have joint pain that I sometimes take medication for

c/ I have occasional joint pain, but it doesn't stop me from doing things

d/ I have no chronic pain, and my bones are strong

How strong is your immune system?

a/ I have a chronic disease, health condition, ongoing infections or an autoimmune condition

b/ I suffer from frequent colds, allergies, viruses or coughs c/ I occasionally suffer colds, coughs or infections

d/ I very rarely get ill and have no allergies or health conditions

How healthy is your heart?

a/ I have high blood pressure and/or a heart condition that I take medication for

b/ I take medication for my heart but don't have a heart condition

c/ I have occasional high blood pressure but am not on medication

d/ I have normal blood pressure and no evidence of heart disease

Feel free to skip to the symptom sections you'd like to address for yourself in Chapter 5

CHAPTER 5:

FEEL BETTER

GET YOUR ENERGY BACK

In health practitioner circles, fatigue is such a common complaint, we have shortened it to 'TATT', meaning 'tired all the time'. It's rare to find a woman content with her energy levels.

Energy is the currency of optimal health. If you're tired, you're more likely to reach for the wrong foods and do less exercise. Your brain isn't going to work as well so you might make poor decisions. Tiredness doesn't promote great relationships and it certainly isn't going to help you be productive, creative or fulfilled in your work.

Many of us tend to accept fatigue as an inevitable part of ageing and a busy or stressful life, but it doesn't have to be that way. Your body is naturally designed to provide you with enough energy for your daily activities, and there might be underlying factors contributing to your exhaustion.

First and foremost, lack of sleep is the primary culprit for feeling tired, so it's essential to rule that out. Beyond that, hormones play a significant role. Take a look at your Feisty Four hormones: excess cortisol will drain your energy, low thyroid hormones can make you feel exhausted, imbalanced blood sugar levels can cause energy dips, and sex hormone fluctuations can disrupt your sleep patterns and leave you feeling fatigued.

Beyond hormones, factors like exposure to toxins, infections, nutrient deficiencies, poor gut health, excessive exercise and underlying health conditions can also contribute to fatigue.

Try these tips, and adopt the EMBRACE protocol in Part 3, however do get checked out or work with a practitioner if your fatigue is persistent or unresolved.

Tips to boost your energy

- **Get enough sleep:** Go to bed earlier and follow my sleep tips (next) to make sure you're getting enough good quality zzzzs.
- **Breathe!** Even if you don't have a lot of time during your day, you can easily do ten deep belly breaths every morning and every night. This can really help reduce your stress hormones and get more oxygen into your cells.
- **Have the right breakfast:** Including protein for breakfast will help stabilise your blood sugar and avoid a mid-morning dip. Or make a quick protein shake with some nut milk and a good quality protein powder. Easy to take with you, filling and nutritious.
- **Reduce your screentime:** There's nothing more tiring than being glued to your laptop, computer or phone! Take regular breaks and try a digital detox once a week.
- **Take a walk:** When your energy is low, take a walk outside, preferably in nature. The daylight, movement and being around greenery will do you wonders.
- **Grab a power nap:** Taking a 10–20-minute power nap has been shown to rejuvenate your energy levels, improving alertness and enhancing performance (especially important if you're not sleeping well at night)
- **Eat energy-producing nutrients:** B vitamins, magnesium, iron, zinc, vitamin C, vitamin E and selenium are all required nutrients to produce energy in your body. These can all be found in vegetables, nuts, seeds, beans/lentils, fish and meat. But you may need to supplement (see Part 3).

> • **Get checked out:** See your doctor to rule out anything more serious that could be related to persistent fatigue. Test your thyroid levels (TSH, T4, T3) and key nutrients including iron, vitamin D, vitamin B12, folate, magnesium – if low, you will need to supplement.

SLEEP LIKE A BABY

Regardless of how healthy your diet and exercise routine may be, if you're not sleeping well, you won't reap the rewards of your efforts. Personally, if I don't get my eight hours a night, I am guaranteed to feel sluggish, unfocused, cranky and craving all the wrong foods (there's a proven link between poor sleep and weight gain).

And if this is an issue for you, you're certainly not alone. Sleep issues are one of the most common complaints for women over 40. According to a 2015 US study, 56% of women over 40 are getting less than the seven hours of sleep per night experts deem restful and healthy.

Sleep is your foundation for healthy ageing. Not only does good sleep make you feel and function better, it's also vital for longevity. While you sleep, your body is hard at work. It's busy repairing any damage done during the day, clearing toxins from the brain, processing key information and memories, strengthening your immune system, regulating your mood, and trying to reduce the risk of health issues such as obesity, heart disease, diabetes, depression, cognitive decline and more.

If you think about it, no other activity delivers so many benefits with so little effort!

However, as we age, our sleep patterns can change, particularly during and after menopause. The decline in oestrogen can affect the production of serotonin, which converts into melatonin, the sleep hormone, while low progesterone means less GABA, your calming neurotransmitter. Night sweats can be another frustrating interruption to your sleep.

Dietary choices also impact sleep; disruptors can include sugar, processed foods, unhealthy fats, alcohol and caffeine. Blood sugar imbalances can lead to those frustrating 3am wake-ups. Dehydration and nutrient deficiencies, including magnesium, tryptophan, B vitamins and vitamin D, can also have a significant impact on sleep.

Your habits and sleep environment can have a significant impact on the quality of your sleep. The sleep-wake cycle is regulated by a group of cells inside the hypothalamus in the brain called the suprachiasmatic nucleus (SCN). The SCN is super sensitive to light signals coming from your eyes. When it's dark, it signals the release of melatonin, your 'sleep hormone', which makes you drowsy. GABA activity increases, making you feel more relaxed and reducing brain activity, while transitioning to slower brain waves that result in non-rapid eye movement (NREM) sleep. Body temperature drops during the evening, further encouraging sleep. When the SCN detects light, it inhibits melatonin production and increases core body temperature to keep us alert and awake.

Cortisol also follows a 24-hour pattern, peaking in the morning and declining throughout the day. However, modern life often disrupts these natural rhythms. Stress can elevate cortisol levels, preventing the body from winding down, while artificial light, especially blue light from screens, confuses the SCN and hinders melatonin production. Irregular sleep schedules and late-night eating further disrupt sleep quality.

Thankfully there's lots you can do to improve your sleep.

Natural ways to sleep better

- **Make sure the room is totally dark:** Blackout blinds are really helpful and try covering up any lights from your alarm clock, TV or gadgets. Try an eye mask and wear blue light blocking glasses if you have to use your laptop, tablet or phone before bed.

- **Keep cool:** Cooler temperatures (aim for 15–19 degrees Celsius) promote the body's natural circadian rhythm and facilitate the release of sleep-inducing hormones, such as melatonin, leading to more restful and rejuvenating sleep.
- **Go to bed earlier:** Try to get to bed before 11pm to maximise the first cycle of deeper non-REM sleep when the body does more of its repair work.
- **Sleep and wake at the same time every day if you can.** This regularity helps the body's sleep-wake cycle
- **Get some daylight:** Get outside every morning to get daylight to stimulate serotonin (or buy a special blue light lamp).
- **Get off the gadgets!** Try to keep your bedroom gadget-free, it will help your brain to switch off.
- **Balance your blood sugar:** Limit quick release carbohydrates like sugar, bread, potatoes, pasta and processed foods, which can disrupt your blood sugar and sleep.
- **Don't eat too late:** Try to stop eating at least two to three hours before bed. Some people do better having a small low-GL snack just before bed (like some nuts or a glass of milk).
- **Get enough magnesium:** Found in dark green leafy veg, whole grains, nuts and seeds, magnesium is your natural relaxant. It can also help with restless legs at night.Magnesium glycinate is my go-to general supplement, but 400–500mg of magnesium threonate can be more effective for sleep.
- **Limit your caffeine:** Try not to consume caffeine past midday if you have trouble sleeping
- **Exercise:** Being physically tired can result in more relaxing sleep at night.
- **Herbal teas:** Try a calming herbal tea before bed. There are many night-time formulas out there, including chamomile, lavender, passionflower and valerian.
- **Calm your mind:** Practise yoga nidra or listen to a mindful meditation before bed.

- **Wear earplugs:** Wax or silicone ear plugs block out noise and reduce the risk of interrupted sleep.
- **Breathwork:** Do a few rounds of box breathing (inhale for four, hold for four, exhale for four, hold for four) until you fall asleep.
- **Write it down:** Keep a notepad by your bed and write down anything that's going around in your head and stopping you sleeping.
- **Avoid the news:** Watching the news or a scary film before bed is going to stress you out, so try to avoid it.
- **Avoid alcohol four to six hours before bed:** It might help you get off to sleep initially, but as alcohol wears off it has a stimulatory effect at about 3am! It may be hard to get back to sleep afterwards.
- **Try body identical HRT**, especially progesterone which can promote a good night's sleep (and reduce anxiety).
- **Take nap snacks:** Long naps will disrupt overnight sleep patterns but taking short (10–20 min) naps can help to mitigate lack of night-time sleep. Get it when you can!

Jump to Part 3, Rest, for more advanced tips and supplements for sleeping better.

BANISH BRAIN FOG AND FORGETFULNESS

Brain fog is one of the biggest things my over-50 friends complain about. The number of times they stop in the middle of a sentence and look around for help – you know, thingummy jig – oh what's his name … arrgggh, it's gone!

Constantly forgetting things or losing your train of thought can be really scary, as it's easy to worry that it's an early sign of Alzheimer's or dementia. There is a key distinction however between occasional forgetfulness and more serious clinical impairment. While this is certainly something to get checked out if you're worried, the good news is that more often than not, it's simply a case of an overburdened brain trying to juggle too many tasks.

Being foggy or forgetful is especially common post menopause, as we know that oestrogen, progesterone and testosterone levels have a protective effect on the brain.

There are other common factors that can be responsible. Stress can damage your brain neurotransmitters, causing mood swings and a lot of foggy thinking. Ever tried to solve a difficult problem when you're stressed out?

Too much sugar or refined carbs can cause damage by promoting oxidative stress, inflammation, and glycation (remember those advanced glycation end-products or AGEs?). These processes can harm cells and tissues in the brain, and disrupt insulin signalling, which is linked to cognitive decline and diseases like Alzheimer's. In fact, type 2 diabetes which is the result of imbalanced blood sugar, almost doubles your risk of dementia.

Nutrient deficiencies, particularly in essential substances like B vitamins, omega-3 fats, iron, protein and antioxidants, can slow down brain cell activity. Blood sugar imbalances, primarily driven by excess insulin from high carb and sugar consumption, can contribute to brain inflammation, disrupting neurotransmitter activity.

Food sensitivities, such as those to wheat, gluten, dairy or soy, can trigger inflammation in the body, including the brain, disrupting nerve signalling. When your microbiome (those trillions of microbes in your gut) is out of balance, you can get brain fog, mood swings, cravings and depression.

Inadequate sleep, even in gradual increments below six hours a night, can significantly impair cognitive functions, memory, focus, reaction time and coordination.

Dehydration is another overlooked factor, as insufficient water intake can reduce cognitive and motor skills, affect memory, focus, brain size, and lead to headaches.

For women over 50, thyroid hormones can be low which can inhibit energy supply to your cells, including brain cells. Typical low thyroid symptoms include memory loss, low mood, fatigue, brain fog, anxiety and low motivation.

Exposure to toxins from various sources, including food, water, household and personal products, over extended periods, can contribute to brain fog, headaches and cognitive decline.

Lastly, a sedentary lifestyle can affect your brain. Physical activity helps to get your blood pumping, delivering oxygen and nutrients to your cells. Your brain needs a lot of both to function well, and if your body isn't moving, your circulation stagnates and so does your brain!

Natural solutions for brain health

- **Nourish your brain cells with:**
  - Oily fish – e.g. salmon, sardines, mackerel, anchovies, rich in EPA and DHA omega-3 fats
  - Healthy fats – avocados, nuts, seeds, olive oil, coconut oil
  - Eggs – rich in choline needed to support methylation
  - Protein – organic grass-fed meat, wild caught fish, organic dairy, soy, quinoa, pulses, beans
  - Antioxidants – colourful fruit and veg (especially berries), dark chocolate, good qualitycoffee. A recent study found that people with Alzheimer's have noticeably lower levels of certain dietary antioxidants, such as lutein, zeaxanthin, and vitamin E in their brains.
  - Herbs and spices – including turmeric, sage, rosemary, clove, cinnamon, oregano, cumin
- **Limit harmful fats** – such as vegetable oils, fried foods, processed foods.
- **Keep hydrated:** Dehydrated brain cells are not going to help clear the fog! It's so important to keep your cells hydrated. That means at least 2L of water (including non-caffeinated drinks) per day for most people, and more if you're exercising.
- **Try a gluten-free diet:** Try a gluten-free diet for three to four weeks and see if your symptoms improve.

- **Balance your blood sugar:** Eat low GL foods, with protein and healthy fats at each meal. Limit snacking.
- **Support your adrenals:** See Part 3 Rest.
- **Reduce exposure to harmful chemicals:** See Part 3 Eliminate.
- **Move more:** Revving up your circulation has proven to be a potent defence against dementia, reducing the risk by up to 30% (and an even more impressive 45% when it comes to Alzheimer's). Jump to Part 3 Move for more on exercise.
- **Get enough sleep:** Follow my sleep tips (in previous section) to make sure you're getting enough good quality zzzzzs.
- **Supplements:** See Part 3 Activate for which supplements to take to support your brain health.

FIND YOUR HAPPY WEIGHT

One of the most common and frustrating menopausal changes for many women is the dreaded 'meno belly'. Out of all the symptoms that accompany this phase of life, it's the extra weight that seems to gather around our midsection that can be the most upsetting.

I'm talking from personal experience here. I've been very open about my lifelong struggles with my weight, something that I had control of during my perimenopause with my nutrition knowledge.

However, in my 50s things changed. I started to accumulate belly fat that just wouldn't shift. I know some of it was down to stress (I was running a very busy business), but it also felt like my body was changing of its own accord!

And here's the reality. Your metabolism is slowing, muscle tissue is decreasing, your fat-*burning* hormones (testosterone, growth hormone, thyroid) are all on the decline, while fat-

storing hormones are dominant (cortisol, insulin). So, it's an UPHILL battle for many women to stave off weight gain.

Like I said in the introduction, I've come to terms with my new postmenopausal body, and I'm now focused on my overall health and muscle strength so I can live longer and better.

However, while acceptance of change is a positive thing, it's important to acknowledge that excess weight poses health risks that you should address where possible. On top of that, excess fat is not harmlessly sitting there, it actually increases inflammation and therefore accelerates ageing.

There are many underlying factors that can affect your weight, so it's worth exploring potential solutions that could make a difference.

Hormones can significantly impact weight management as they are responsible for regulating your metabolism, appetite, blood sugar and your weight. Any imbalance can cause weight gain.

Cortisol likes to store fat around the middle, with four times more cortisol receptors around your belly area than anywhere else. When stress levels are high, cortisol stimulates appetite, making us crave sugar and carbs, which are stored as fat if not used for energy. Cortisol also breaks down muscle and slows metabolism, making it harder to burn fat.

Insulin is known as the 'fat-storing' hormone, as it stores excess glucose in fat cells. The more insulin produced, the more fat is stored, leading to a cycle of cravings for carbs and sugar that is especially challenging to control post menopause.

Thyroid hormones regulate metabolism, so any deficiency can make weight loss difficult without extreme dieting. And declining oestrogen and progesterone levels during menopause affect how we handle carbohydrates and regulate metabolism and fat distribution.

Other hormones such as leptin, ghrelin and cholecystokinin (CCK) are also important in regulating appetite and weight. Ghrelin stimulates hunger, while leptin and CCK signal to the brain that you're full. As we get older, hormonal changes can disrupt the balance between these hormones, leading to increased appetite and decreased metabolism, which can contribute to weight gain. Additionally, menopause and the accumulation of fat can make us more prone to leptin resistance, which can stop the 'full' signal to the brain, making it easy to overeat.

What else can impact your weight? As well as the right balance of exercise, we know that sleep deprivation increases production of your hunger hormone ghrelin. Even your gut has a role to play by influencing how your body absorbs nutrients, regulates appetite and manages inflammation.

Addressing all these underlying issues however may provide a better outcome for you than just focusing on your diet.

Tips for better weight management

- **Increase protein:** Protein helps with satiety, building muscle, boosting metabolism, regulating appetite hormones, stabilising blood sugar levels and enhancing insulin sensitivity, all factors that help you manage your weight.
- **Reduce hidden sugars:** You're probably minimising sugar, but did you know that carbohydrates are just long sugars? And fruit is still sugar? And alcohol is mainly sugar? Have you checked the labels of your favourite sauces, dressings,ready meals, 'protein bars' for added sugar? Did you knowthat a baguette has a higher glycaemic load than white table sugar? Avoid artificial sweeteners such as sucralose and aspartame, which can disrupt blood sugar and gut function.

- **Balance your blood sugar:** Blood sugar dips and spikes can cause cravings for more sugar/carbs, and keep you in fat storing mode. Make sure your meals have sufficient protein,healthy fats and complex carbs, including fibre to slow down glucose release.
- **Stop the calorie-controlled diets**: Many diets are based on calorie restriction, which can force the body into survival mode, slowing down your metabolism and speeding up your cravings. NOT a sustainable way to keep the pounds off.
- **Ditch the alcohol:** As well as a hidden sugar source, alcohol disrupts your blood sugar and your willpower!
- **Fasting:** Overnight fasting or Time Restricted Eating is one of the easiest ways to manage your weight if you're suited to it. Jump to Part 3 Activate for more on this.
- **Limit snacking:** If you are snacking between meals, the body is constantly using up your sugar stores as energy and doesn't always get around to burning fat stores. Leaving four to six hours between meals can help the body burn those fat stores for energy.
- **Hydrate:** Dehydration can be mistaken for hunger. Drink a glass of water before food to make sure!
- **Emotional eating:** It's common to reach for food if we're sad, stressed, lonely, uncomfortable or bored. Increasing awareness of WHY we're eating can help work out what to do instead. Keep a food and symptom journal (or app) to spot any patterns.
- **Portion control:** Sometimes we are eating really healthy foods, and not realising we're just eating too much of them. Nut butter may be nutritious, but a whole jar of it will not help you lose weight! Watch your portion sizes, eat slowly and stop eating before you feel 100% full.
- **Take 1 tbsp apple cider vinegar before meals:** Research has shown that this can reduce your weight without making any other changes.
- **Sleep:** Poor sleep can increase your hunger hormone ghrelin, plus you're more likely to reach for the carbs if you're tired and groggy.

- **Exercise:** Getting the right exercise balance is key. Sitting all day causes your body to slow your metabolism, and there are no signals to your fat cells to burn fat. Over-exercising can also be a cause of weight loss resistance ironically. Doing too much can raise cortisol – and signals the body hangs on to fat.
- **Stress management:** Cortisol loves to store belly fat. Switching off your stress response daily will help to minimise this.
- **Check your thyroid:** Get your thyroid tested to rule out deficiency.
- **Gut health:** Looking after your gut can really help manage your weight.

Following the EMBRACE protocol in Part 3 will help you find a healthy weight (and a level of self-acceptance of your changing body shape if necessary).

RELIEVE ANXIETY AND BALANCE YOUR MOOD

I had hoped that things had changed since I was offered antidepressants for my mood swings and anxiety in my 40s, but I'm still hearing similar stories every single day from women in our clinic. Don't get me wrong, these and other medications can be a lifesaver for many women, but I don't believe they should be considered as first-line treatment for menopause.

While extreme mood swings (and often pure rage) might be more common as you go through perimenopause, once you get past menopause, the extremes can often settle into more of a low-grade depression. Sometimes it can just feel like a kind of numbness or inability to feel joy or excitement about anything. Or you may still carry the rage that is always there under the surface.

Maybe you find you're more anxious post menopause, even if you have never had anxiety in the past. Physical symptoms can go along with these feelings, including sweating, palpitations, panic attacks, shaking, nausea and diarrhoea being just a few.

Nobody can be happy and calm all the time, but understanding some of the underlying factors at play can empower you to make substantial improvements in how you feel.

Physical imbalances
Brain chemicals, or neurotransmitters, such as serotonin (the 'happy' hormone), dopamine (the 'feel-good' hormone), adrenaline, GABA (the 'calming' hormone), glutamate and acetylcholine, are crucial to how you feel, think and behave. Your brain must maintain a delicate balance to keep these neurotransmitters in check. They transmit messages between neurons, creating a complex communication system responsible for the thousands of thoughts, emotions and sensations you experience daily.

Hormones and the brain share a strong and complex relationship, where signals determine which hormones are produced, and these hormones, in turn, influence brain activity and mental health. Oestrogen plays a vital role in mood and anxiety regulation, especially during and after menopause, with lower levels potentially leading to decreased serotonin and GABA activity, resulting in mood swings, depression and anxiety. Progesterone has a calming effect by stimulating GABA receptors, so when levels decline, mood and sleep can be negatively impacted. Testosterone also affects the brain, with low levels leading to reduced mood, motivation and increased anxiety.

High (or low) cortisol levels interfere with neurotransmitters like serotonin, dopamine and GABA, while low thyroid hormones can cause depression, anxiety, brain fog and memory loss. Additionally, menopause increases susceptibility to insulin resistance, leading to more inflammation in the brain, altering neurotransmitters and impacting mood.

Nutrient deficiencies
There are key vitamins and minerals that are crucial for brain health. Magnesium is often referred to as nature's tranquiliser, relaxing the body and muscles and helping with stress. Vitamins D, B6 and B12 help modulate serotonin and other neurotransmitters in the brain. B12, B6 and folate are vital for methylation processes and along with iron help oxygenate

the brain and produce serotonin and dopamine. Omega-3 fats and zinc are key to supporting brain cell health. If we don't get enough of these key nutrients from our diet, OR we are not absorbing them very well, deficiencies can occur and cause mood and anxiety issues.

Gut-brain

The gut-brain connection refers to the direct line of communication between your gut and brain, acting like a highway where signals are exchanged between the two. Your gut makes the majority of your serotonin, a key player in controlling your mood. When the balance of bacteria in this community is disrupted, it can potentially result in feelings of low mood or anxiety. This is why keeping your gut happy with good nutrition is vital for your physical AND mental health (more on that later in Part 2 and Part 3, Eliminate).

Emotional health

There are many therapies that can help you manage your emotional state. Talking therapies or counselling offer a supportive, non-judgmental environment to explore thoughts, feelings and behaviours. Many therapists use CBT (Cognitive Behavioural Therapy) to identify and challenge negative thought patterns contributing to anxiety or mood issues, providing coping skills and techniques such as relaxation exercises and problem-solving strategies. Hypnotherapy can address issues like anxiety, phobias, trauma, pain management and habits such as smoking cessation or weight loss. Mindfulness and meditation practices are also effective at calming the mind, focusing on the present moment and cultivating gratitude and positive thoughts.

Jump to Connect (Self) in Part 3 for more on emotional health.

Tips to improve your mood or anxiety

- **Manage your stress:** Prioritise switch-off time every day to balance your cortisol levels (more on this in Part 3 Rest).

- **Balance your blood sugar:** Limit the risk of insulin resistance impacting your brain by eating protein and healthy fats at each meal with plenty of vegetables and fibre. Limit sugar, alcohol, caffeine and refined carbs. Avoid snacking between meals if you can.
- **Move more:** Exercise helps to improve mood and stress levels. But find the right balance for you, don't be too sedentary but don't over-exercise either – that can be detrimental if you don't have the energy reserves. Do what feels good.
- **Get your morning daylight:** Morning light is rich in blue light wavelengths that not only help to reset your body clock each day but also trigger the production of serotonin. It's like a daily dose of good vibes sent straight from the sun (even if it's cloudy!). A walk in nature fulfils your daylight, move and stress management needs.
- **Eat brain-healthy foods:** Including oats, brown rice, quinoa, eggs, turkey, dark chocolate, nuts, seeds, seafood, oily fish and dark green leafy veg.
- **Look after your gut:** Eliminate foods that you might be sensitive to (e.g. gluten or dairy) for a few weeks to notice how you feel. Try foods rich in probiotics such as live yoghurt, sauerkraut, kefir, kombucha to rebalance your gut bacteria.
- **Try body identical HRT:** If your symptoms are caused by low levels of oestrogen and progesterone, hormone replacement can be really helpful
- **Include phytoestrogen foods:** If you're not on HRT, including phytoestrogens in your diet can help regulate your sex hormone levels, e.g. organic soy, flaxseeds, lentils.
- **Supplements:** Add in some mood-enhancing nutrients including:
  - **A good multivitamin** – with methylated B vitamins (B6, folate and B12) – needed for neurotransmitter function, as well as key minerals needed for brain cells (including zinc)

- **Omega fats** – EPA, DHA and GLA – your brain is made up of 60% fat
- **Magnesium** – can help with stress and improve brain plasticity
- **Vitamin D** – can help to reduce inflammation and regulate nerve cell function
- **5-HTP** can be helpful for low moods (do not take if you're already taking an antidepressant). It contains tryptophan – an amino acid that is a precursor to serotonin
- **Adrenal formulas,** including rhodiola, ashwagandha, Holy Basil, ginseng, Schisandra, Shatavari
- **CBD** – cannabidiol, derived directly from the hemp plant – while it's a cousin of marijuana, it's non-addictive and very safe, and can help with stress, anxiety, mood and sleep
- **Try talking therapy,** counselling, CBT or hypnotherapy: practitioner if you're new to these therapies.
- **Testing:** If you can, get yourself properly tested – hormones, gut health, vitamins and minerals all have an impact on our mental health and brain function (if nothing else, get your thyroid, vitamin D and B12 tested – they can be easily overlooked).

INTIMATE REGIONS

There are some postmenopausal challenges that are still very much in the taboo cupboard. For far too long, advice and support for women on these issues has been scant, but we're addressing them head-on right here.

It was only in 2014 that the health authorities finally recognised the range of symptoms that affect our genital and urinary systems during and post menopause. They called it GSM, or Genitourinary Syndrome of Menopause (catchy!).

In recent large cohort studies, nearly two thirds of the women who were postmenopausal reported suffering uncomfortable symptoms in their vulva-vaginal area.

The most talked about issue? Vaginal dryness. But that wasn't all; they also mentioned painful sex, irritation, itching, tenderness, leakage, urgency, infections and even spotting or bleeding during intimacy.

The truth is that oestrogen is like a wonder worker for our whole pelvic region, keeping the vulva, vagina and lower urinary tract happy and working properly. Declining oestrogen can cause a ripple effect of symptoms, some irritating and others downright painful, affecting everything from our day-to-day comfort to our sexual wellbeing.

Unlike hot flushes and night sweats which usually get better as time goes by, the issues affecting our intimate areas can linger — and even get worse if they go untreated. While they aren't usually dangerous, they can really take a toll on our intimate relationships and overall quality of life.

Let's have a look into some of these:

Vaginal dryness (or atrophy)
Possibly the most common symptom that can start in perimenopause and endure well beyond. Oestrogen helps to keep the walls of the vagina thick, elastic and well-lubricated. When levels go down during menopause, the tissues in the vagina don't get as much nourishment and support as they used to, so they can get thinner, dryer and less flexible.

Irritation, itching or burning
As the tissue around the vulva and vagina becomes more fragile, it can cause irritation and discomfort. You might notice increased sensitivity, constant itching or a burning sensation that can be quite distressing. Itching or soreness around the urethra and anus is also quite common. These symptoms can occasionally be signs of something more serious, so it's important to get checked out by your doctor if they persist.

Painful sex
If you have dryness or irritation inside or around the vagina, penetrative sex can be very painful. Before I started taking HRT,

I experienced this and it felt like being impaled by a hot poker! This can obviously have a huge impact on your sexual desire and relationship with your partner.

Bladder health and urinary tract infections (UTIs)

Oestrogen helps to keep the lining of the bladder and the urethra healthy. When there's less of it around, these tissues can become thinner and more fragile, which unfortunately makes them more susceptible to UTIs, the most common of which is cystitis. Changes in vaginal pH and microbiome that can also happen as a result of declining oestrogen can further increase the risk of UTIs as well as bacterial vaginosis, which can cause unusual discharge, a fishy odour, itching and discomfort. Do get checked out if you have these symptoms.

Leaking, urgency or incontinence

A whole industry has flourished targeting women who experience embarrassing leaking (you know the ads I'm referring to!). But it's not something that we should accept as 'normal'. Lower oestrogen levels can affect your bladder's ability to stretch to hold urine and then contract to release it, which can cause an increased urgency to pee or the uncomfortable experience of bladder leakage. However, there are solutions. Using localised oestrogen treatment, and/or strengthening your pelvic floor, can offer significant improvements.

Pelvic organ prolapse

Declining oestrogen can weaken the muscles and tissues that support the pelvic region, and this can cause the dropping or descent of the pelvic organs (usually the bladder, uterus or rectum). Other factors can contribute to the risk of prolapse, including a history of vaginal childbirth, obesity, chronic coughing or issues with chronic constipation. It might manifest as a feeling of heaviness or pulling in the pelvis, and in some cases, it might even be visible or palpable in the vaginal canal.

Engaging in pelvic floor exercises, maintaining a healthy weight, and seeking medical advice early on can be your allies in preventing and managing prolapse. There are various treatments available, including physiotherapy and, in more severe cases, surgery, to help manage this condition and maintain your quality of life.

Hard to achieve or lower intensity orgasms
Oestrogen has been nourishing and taking care of your vaginal tissue's elasticity and lubrication for years. When levels dip, you might find the road to orgasm can be a bit longer and possibly requiring a more scenic route. Physical sensations might change due to alterations in the vaginal tissue and reduced blood flow to the area, and hormonal shifts can also alter your emotional responses during intimacy, adding a different feel to the overall experience.

It's vital that as soon as you notice any symptoms discussed in this chapter, you should contact your doctor to get checked out. There are many different medical treatments that could help, depending on the diagnosis.

HRT is one of the more obvious treatments. According to studies, when systemic (body identical) HRT is used to treat other menopausal symptoms, vaginal symptoms are generally improved as well. However, in around 10–15% of women, systemic HRT doesn't resolve vaginal symptoms, and additional low-dose vaginal oestrogen may be needed.

If you can't or don't want to take systemic HRT, then local vaginal oestrogen therapy (oestrogen pessaries, creams or a vaginal ring) can be an effective and safe way to relieve symptoms for many women, including women who have had breast cancer.

Let's talk about sex
If you're suffering any of the symptoms relating to GSM, sex is going to be the last thing on your mind. Even if you don't have these symptoms, there are many other factors that can affect your libido. In fact, studies have shown 75% of women over 40 feel like their sex drive is decreasing.

Oestrogen is the hormone that makes you feel sexy (it's there to make babies), so when levels decline, it's not surprising your desire can go down along with it. Progesterone is your anti-stress hormone, and along with testosterone, helps to maintain your sex drive.

Stress and sex? They really don't go together! When you're in survival mode, the body is not going to be diverting essential resources to your libido for reproduction. So cortisol dampens down your sex hormones, making you more likely to reach for a chocolate bar instead of your partner.

Thyroid hormones regulate sex hormone production and help convert cholesterol into progesterone, so if your thyroid levels are low, your sex drive may plummet, leaving you feeling tired rather than sexy.

Certain medications (including the birth control pill, some forms of HRT and antidepressants) can include side effects that affect your libido. If you suspect this may be the case for you, do discuss alternatives with your doctor.

The good news is, recognising GSM symptoms is the first step to finding relief. Whether it's through medical treatments, diet, lifestyle or supplements, there are ways to reclaim your comfort and sexual desire (if required!).

Natural solutions to relieve GSM

- **Diet:** Eat plenty of healthy fats (for sex hormones and lubrication), colourful veg, garlic (antimicrobial), stay hydrated and avoid food stressors (including alcohol). Including phytoestrogen foods can help with some symptoms (including organic soy, flaxseeds, red clover extract).
- **Relax:** Make sure you take some time for yourself, whatever your commitments are. Try mindfulness, acupuncture, massage or other relaxation techniques. Do something you love every day – walking in nature, reading, massage, talking to a good friend, watching a funny movie or taking a warm bath in Epsom salts.

- **Lubricants, moisturisers and non-toxic personal care:** Avoid products with chemicals in them that could irritate your skin. There are many brands that use non-toxic ingredients that are safe.
- **Exercise:** Exercise stimulates circulation, blood flow and oxygen to all the right parts. So, make sure you get out walking, do some yoga, Pilates, weights – whatever makes you happy. But don't over-exercise because that's another stress that's likely to kill your libido.
- **Pelvic floor support:** Having a strong pelvic floor is like having a solid foundation for a building; it holds everything together and keeps it in place. It can help prevent issues such as urinary incontinence and pelvic organ prolapse, as well as enhance sexual pleasure. Do regular 'Kegel' type exercises or find a specialist pelvic floor physiotherapist or yoga class.
- **Talk to your partner:** Explain what's happening to your body during this stage. If your partner can understand, they are more likely to be able to help and support you through the worst of it. If that isn't enough, counselling may be helpful or maybe consult a sex therapist.
- **Check yourself:** Get a handheld mirror and check yourself regularly. Don't self-diagnose. Any changes (e.g. redness, sores, marks, discharge, moles), book in to see your GP (you can ask for a female doctor if you feel uncomfortable).

- **Supplements:** There are certain supplements I'd recommend to help with genital and urinary health:
  - Omega-7 sea buckthorn oil – this can help with dryness
  - Omega-3 EPA and DHA. Look for good brands with at least 1000mg of combined EPA/DHA
  - A good multivitamin will give you the basic vitamins and minerals you need
  - Maca is 'nature's Viagra'! The right forms of maca can help with energy, stamina and libido
  - D-Mannose, cranberry and vitamin C – for recurrent UTIs (including cystitis)

- L-Arginine – might help stimulate nitric oxide to boost blood flow to genital organs, and is naturally antimicrobial
- Probiotics – Lactobacillus strains can help balance and restore the vaginal microbiome
- **Body identical HRT:** Natural forms of oestrogen, progesterone and/or testosterone can help with some of these issues. Discuss with your doctor.

HAPPY GUT, HAPPY YOU

Having worked with women's hormones for over ten years, I've witnessed the prevalence of gut and digestive issues, particularly among women approaching or experiencing menopause.

Issues, ranging from constipation to heartburn, are common but only part of the picture. An unhappy gut can manifest symptoms throughout the body, including headaches, joint pain, gum disease, depression, anxiety, brain fog, mood swings, fatigue, weight gain, poor sleep, sinusitis, asthma and autoimmune conditions like psoriasis, rheumatoid arthritis, and coeliac disease, among others.

Whether you've been diagnosed with IBS or you're just suffering with some of these symptoms, you may feel like that's your lot, and that you've got to put up with it for the rest of your life.

That's because there's no effective cure in the medical world. IBS is not even a disease, it's actually a collection of symptoms unrelated to recognised conditions like bowel cancer or inflammatory bowel disease.

Even if you are diagnosed with IBS, you're pretty much left to manage it on your own. There are some drugs that can help with symptoms, but they're doing just that, focusing on symptom management rather than addressing the underlying cause.

Fortunately, if you can pinpoint the root cause, there's a real chance of resolving the issue once and for all.

Underlying infections or microbial imbalances
We have a whole ecosystem living in our intestines, around 100 trillion (or thereabouts!) different species of microbes and organisms that are vital for our wellbeing. They have a whole host of roles to play, and their balance can be disrupted by factors such as infection, stress, diet, medications and toxins.

One of the hardest to diagnose conditions is SIBO (Small Intestine Bacterial Overgrowth). It's a condition associated with excess microbes, usually bacteria or fungi, in the small intestine rather than colon. It comes with bloating, distention, gas and/or crampy pain. It's not often recognised or diagnosed in the medical world (often just put down to IBS), but specialists can test for it and treat it.

Another often underdiagnosed infection is caused by *Helicobacter pylori* (*H. Pylori* for short). This is a very common bacterium that lives in the stomach. It's harmless for most of us, but for about 14% of people, it can cause pain and inflammation (gastritis), and if left untreated can lead to stomach ulcers and a higher risk of stomach cancer. It's even been linked to Alzheimer's disease. If you're experiencing stomach issues and haven't been tested for it yet, it's worth discussing with your doctor as it's easily testable and treatable.

Low stomach acid or enzymes
Hydrochloric acid and digestive enzymes are produced in your stomach to help break down your food and pass it down the system. If food is not digested properly due to insufficient gastric secretions, it can sit in the gut too long, potentially resulting in gas, bloating and indigestion. Problems here can also result in further gastrointestinal issues, such as Helicobacter pylori infection, dysbiosis, food allergies and intolerances, rheumatoid arthritis, acne rosacea, asthma, and

reduced secretion of intrinsic factor, which is necessary for vitamin B12 absorption. Natural supplements can effectively support stomach acid and enzymes to provide relief.

Food sensitivities

Certain foods can trigger an autoimmune response. This is not immediately dangerous (like an allergy) but can cause a lot of symptoms and over time can damage your gut lining. The most common ones are gluten and dairy, although any foods can cause a reaction if your gut is inflamed and sensitive.

Leaky gut

The medical name for a leaky gut is 'intestinal impermeability'. Imagine your gut lining looks like a colander instead of a tight sieve. Being more porous can allow waste particles, undigested food, pathogens and toxins to leak through the digestive tract into the bloodstream. This can trigger a reaction from your immune system, because it doesn't recognise these things as normal, which in turn can cause inflammation, and increase the risk of autoimmune conditions like rheumatoid arthritis, lupus, type 1 diabetes, Hashimoto's or Graves' disease, coeliac disease, Crohn's disease, psoriasis, MS, among others.

Stress

We all know that stress can mess with our bowel habits. When the body is in fight-or-flight mode, the last thing you need to do is digest your lunch. If we're constantly stressed, this can result in long-term gut issues.

Poor diet

Refined carbohydrates and sugars in your diet are favourite foods for bad bacteria and yeast, which can build up in your gut and cause an imbalance in your microbiome.

While many of these causal factors are diet or lifestyle related, there can be more serious conditions that you need to rule out with your doctor if you've had prolonged and/or unexplained symptoms. These include coeliac disease, Crohn's disease, ulcerative colitis, gastric ulcers, appendicitis, gallstones and certain cancers. Get checked if you're worried.

IBD (inflammatory bowel disease) is a chronic condition that affects the digestive tract and can cause some serious discomfort. It comes in two main forms: Crohn's disease and ulcerative colitis. These conditions involve inflammation and damage to the lining of the intestines, leading to symptoms like abdominal pain, diarrhoea, fatigue and weight loss. The exact cause of IBD is still not fully understood, but researchers believe it's a combination of genetic factors, environmental triggers and an abnormal immune response.

There are medications that help manage symptoms but diet and lifestyle can also make a big difference too. Certain foods can trigger flare-ups, so it's important to identify and avoid your personal trigger foods. Additionally, including anti-inflammatory foods like fruits, vegetables, whole foods and healthy fats can be beneficial.

Stress has been known to worsen symptoms, so finding things that help you relax and unwind can make a world of difference. And don't forget the importance of getting enough rest and sleep to support your body's healing process.

In Part 3 Eliminate, we will look at more strategies on how to look after your gut health, liver and immune system.

Tips to support your gut

- **Eat slowly:** How many times do we bolt our food down, especially when we're busy? Just set aside 10 to 15 minutes to eat more mindfully. The first stage of digestion is in the mouth, so chew slowly to get your saliva flowing and stimulate the production of stomach acid and enzymes.
- **Stimulate your juices!** Take some betaine HCL and/or digestive enzymes to stimulate your gastric juices and digest your food properly. Alternatively, a teaspoon of apple cider vinegar before meals can help. (Do not do this if you have acid reflux or any stomach conditions.)

- **Stress management:** Set aside at least ten minutes to yourself every day to do some deep breathing, mindfulness or meditation, or whatever it is that switches off your stress response.
- **Keep a food and symptom diary:** Try to spot any patterns between what you eat and how you feel.
- **Remove the food triggers:** Remove any potential triggers (starting with gluten and dairy) for a minimum of three weeks, then re-introduce them one by one. You'll soon notice any reactions.
- **Clean up your diet:** Eat whole real foods, avoid processed foods and refined carbs, and make sure you're piling on a good variety of vegetables.
- **Certain medications** can be problematic for the gut. This includes painkillers like ibuprofen and paracetamol which can damage your gut lining. Antibiotics can strip out all your bacteria, good and bad, so try to take a good-quality probiotic supplement alongside or after your course, and take them at night so that you're not competing with the medication.
- **Fibre:** Feed your good bacteria with plenty of fibre (they love it!). Include pulses, seeds, whole grains, fruit and plenty of different coloured vegetables if these foods are well tolerated.
- **Probiotic foods:** Including live yoghurt, sauerkraut, kefir, kombucha, miso and kimchi.
- **Prebiotic foods:** Eat foods that feed your good bacteria, including leeks, onions, garlic, green bananas and cold cooked potatoes.
- **Limit alcohol:** Alcohol can damage your gut lining. Remove or reduce your alcohol intake, and always have it with food.
- **Stay active:** Exercise helps to keep the bowels working.
- **Look after your mouth:** Don't forget that your mouth is part of your GI tract so keep it healthy.
- **Supplements** can help. Magnesium citrate relaxes bowel muscles (great if you're constipated), digestive enzymes, fish oils help to reduce inflammation, probiotics and vitamin D to help regulate your immune system.

> • **Identify any infections:** Private stool testing can identify underlying gut infections or imbalances that could be causing your symptoms. Ask your doctor for an H. pylori test if you have stomach issues.

HEALTHY JOINTS AND BONES

Maintaining healthy joints and bones is something you need to be prioritising now if you want to stay mobile and independent for this next chapter of your life.

Joint health

Joint pain can make you feel old overnight, but it's not something you have to simply accept as a part of ageing. By understanding the underlying causes and implementing proactive strategies, you can significantly improve your joint health and maintain an active, pain-free lifestyle.

Aside from occasional achy joints, certain medical conditions, such as arthritis, can become more prevalent as we age. Osteoarthritis is due to the breakdown of the cartilage that acts as a cushion and shock absorber for the joints, whereas rheumatoid arthritis is an autoimmune disease that affects the membranes surrounding your joints. Autoimmune conditions usually develop from inflammation in the gut, so improving your gut health is often helpful.

We also know that hormones play a vital role in joint health, so it's not surprising that many women start to report joint pain in their 40s and 50s as oestrogen levels start to decline, stress levels increase and thyroid conditions are more common.

Oestrogen helps reduce inflammation, the main cause of joint pain and swelling. It helps to increase bone production and regulate fluid levels in your body, reducing oedema and swelling around joints. Oestrogen can also modulate pain perception, threshold and tolerance by interacting with neurotransmitters such as serotonin, dopamine and norepinephrine.

Excess cortisol can stimulate pro-inflammatory cytokines, and inhibit muscle, cartilage and bone production, while low thyroid hormones can reduce cartilage integrity and lubrication, leading to symptoms such as stiffness, pain and decreased mobility.

While there are genetic considerations to both diagnosed arthritis and general joint pain, other considerations include injury, poor posture, wear and tear and musculoskeletal issues.

Fortunately, many of these factors can be influenced through diet, lifestyle changes and inflammation management, which will be discussed in more detail in Part 3.

Bone health

If your joints are the key to movement and flexibility, then your bones are the solid structure that hold you up. And they need to be strong as you get older to avoid osteoporosis and fractures.

The stats for osteoporosis are scary – worldwide 1 in 3 women over 50 will suffer an osteoporotic fracture (1 in 5 for men). And it's risky. Research suggests you've got a 1 in 5 chance of dying within a year following a hip fracture.

I guess my mum was lucky. Fifteen years ago, in her early 60s, she was in a supermarket car park ready to do her weekly shop. She opened her door and as she went to get out of the car, her foot caught in her seat belt, and she fell from the car seat onto the ground. Now, she has a Mini, so it wasn't far to fall (about a foot!) but it smashed her hip into lots of tiny pieces.

It was only after her operation, and subsequent new hip, that she was diagnosed with osteoporosis. There were no symptoms that alerted her, and she had never had a bone scan. It took a nasty hip fracture to find out.

Unfortunately she's not alone. Hip fractures occupy more beds in Western hospitals than any other disease, with deaths occurring as a result of complications such as pneumonia, blood clots or other medical issues stemming from the fracture or its treatment.

Osteoporosis literally means 'porous bones'. Your bone is living tissue, an active endocrine organ. It's constantly being built and destroyed, and as we get older it's this balance that, if it's upset, can cause more destruction than new build, leaving your bones weak and brittle, and easily broken.

Oestrogen helps to regulate bone remodelling, a continuous process of bone formation and resorption. Declining levels can lead to a loss of bone density and an increased risk of osteoporosis.

Bone health is usually measured by bone mineral density or BMD, measured by a DEXA scan – which you can get on the NHS once you hit 65. But if you're over 50 and are at increased risk of osteoporosis, you may want to consider going privately.

Osteopenia is the first stage, where BMD is lower than it should be but not low enough to be osteoporotic. Osteoporosis is where the BMD has decreased significantly, and risk of fracture is high.

The first step is to be aware of the risk factors so you can manage them. Of course, age, menopause and genetics are the biggest, but your diet and lifestyle play a vital role too. Nutritional deficiencies can contribute to poor joint and bone health, notably vitamin D, magnesium, boron, vitamin K2, calcium, strontium, molybdenum, manganese and phosphorus.

Additionally, a lack of weight-bearing exercise, smoking, excessive alcohol consumption and the intake of fizzy drinks and caffeine can further increase the risk of joint pain and bone loss. Diets high in animal protein or dairy, particularly if derived from non-organic sources, may have also have a detrimental effect for some women, while gluten sensitivity or coeliac disease can impair gut health and nutrient absorption, further increasing the risk of osteoporosis. It is also crucial to address chronic inflammation, as it can accelerate joint pain and bone destruction.

Fortunately, there are many things you can do to support your joints and bones as you get older.

Ways to naturally support your joints and bones:

- **Adopt a low GL diet:** Switch from white carbs to wholegrains, eat plenty of healthy fats and protein at each meal, reduce sugar, caffeine, fizzy drinks and alcohol.
- **Add anti-inflammatory foods to your diet:** Oily fish, nuts, seeds (especially flax and chia), fruit, veg, spices. Turmeric can help with inflammation and pain. Montmorency cherry juice can also help those with arthritic pain.
- **Reduce processed foods, vegetable oils, dairy and processed meat,** in favour of more plant foods.
- **Try an elimination diet:** Gluten, dairy, soy, eggs, corn, yeast are the main culprits that can increase inflammation if you're sensitive. Go without for at least three weeks and see if symptoms improve.
- **Stay hydrated:** Drink plenty of water throughout your day.
- **Stop smoking:** Smoking reduces bone density, impairing calcium absorption, disrupting hormone levels and increasing the risk of fractures due to decreased bone strength and other associated factors.
- **Manage your stress levels:** Try deep belly breathing, reading, meditation, music, nature, warm baths, sleep.
- **Weight-bearing exercise:** Walking, jogging, resistance or weight training – all great for increasing blood flow to joints and bones.
- **Improve your balance, posture and mobility:** Pilates, yoga, balance work will help you avoid and recover from falls.

- **Body identical HRT:** If you're able to replace the hormones that protect your joints and bones, then do. Alternatively, **phytoestrogens can help balance oestrogen** – the biggest sources are organic soy, flaxseeds, red clover, sage, hops, black cohosh.
- **Supplements:** Helpful supplements include magnesium (in oil form you can rub into the skin around the joint area), vitamin D3 with K2, omega-3 EPA/DHA, glucosamine, isoflavones, turmeric, collagen.

STRENGTHEN YOUR IMMUNE SYSTEM

Your immune system is intricate and complex – and incredibly busy. Every day, it faces a barrage of microbes from our surroundings, including the air we breathe, the food we consume and the products we interact with.

A less-than-optimal immune system can manifest in a variety of ways, impacting different bodily systems and contributing to a range of health issues. Here are some of the common signs, symptoms and conditions that may suggest your immune system isn't working as efficiently as it could be:

- **Frequent infections:** such as colds and sinus infections, or skin infections.
- **Prolonged illness:** when it takes you longer than usual to recover from minor illnesses.
- **Fatigue:** persistent fatigue is more than just tiredness; it can be a sign that your body is working overtime to combat threats it might normally brush off easily.
- **Digestive issues:** regular issues like diarrhoea, constipation, bloating and gas can indicate an imbalance in gut flora, which in turn can weaken the immune system.
- **Food intolerances:** sensitivities to certain foods (such as gluten or dairy) can lead to chronic inflammation, a considerable stressor on the immune system.

- **Skin problems:** such as eczema, psoriasis or frequent rashes.
- **Poor wound healing:** if it takes a long time for wounds or cuts to heal, it's another signal that your immune system might not be operating optimally.
- **Frequent allergies or asthma:** often the result of an overactive immune system, which ends up attacking harmless particles like pollen, mould or dust.
- **Cancer:** your immune system is key to controlling the build-up and growth of cancer cells in the body. When the immune system is weakened or compromised, it may fail to recognise and effectively target cancer cells, allowing them to proliferate and form tumours. And it may struggle to control the spread of cancer cells to other parts of the body, a process known as metastasis.

Autoimmune conditions

Autoimmune conditions occur when the immune system attacks healthy cells, mistaking them for foreign invaders. Such mutiny is usually down to a culmination of factors including genetics, stress, gut health, hormonal imbalances and unfortunately your gender (70% of all autoimmune conditions affect women). Hormone changes in menopause can switch on the inflammatory response and in some people, excess antibody production. Other risk factors include genetics, diet, toxins, stress and gut health.

There are over 80 different types of known autoimmune conditions and they often come in clusters, meaning if you have one type of autoimmune condition then you might be prone to developing more. Various body systems can be affected, including the thyroid (e.g. Hashimoto's and Graves' disease), skin (e.g. psoriasis), joints (e.g. rheumatoid arthritis), hormones (e.g. type 1 diabetes, endometriosis), hair (e.g. alopecia) and gut (e.g. coeliac disease). Or multiple organ systems such as lupus.

Supporting your immune system and gut with diet, lifestyle and supplements can help to improve your resilience and reduce risk of autoimmune conditions.

Natural ways to support your immune system

- **Diet:** A nutrient-dense, anti-inflammatory, antioxidant rich diet can be helpful in reducing inflammation and supporting your gut and immune function. If you have an autoimmune condition, you may need to eliminate common trigger foods such as gluten and dairy and try bone broth and collagen to heal the gut lining. Probiotic rich foods, such as fermented vegetables and kefir, can help to support gut health and improve immune function. Limit foods that can promote inflammation and oxidative stress, such as sugar, refined carbs, processed foods, vegetable oils and alcohol.
- **Reduce toxins:** Use natural household and personal products, avoid pesticides and other chemicals in food, limit plastics and filter your water. Exercise, heat therapy, massage and adequate hydration are great ways to support your liver and natural detoxification pathways.
- **Manage stress:** Chronic stress and cortisol weaken your immune function and can lead to inflammation and immune dysregulation.
- **Sleep:** When your body rests and repairs, it releases proteins called cytokines while you're asleep, which help fight infection and inflammation. Make sure you are prioritising sleep as much as possible.
- **Move:** Consistent exercise helps to reduce inflammation and increase your immune protection cells.
- **Rebalance your microbiome:** You can take a good quality probiotic, but it's best to invest in a comprehensive stool test to investigate any specific underlying infections that could be triggering the immune system (e.g. bacteria, virus, yeast, parasite).
- **Supplement:** These vitamins and minerals play various roles in supporting the immune system. They act as antioxidants, shielding against harmful reactive oxygen species and aiding in the growth and functionality of immune cells

- Vitamin D – your key immune defender! Make sure you're supplementing at least 2000IU per day during the winter, but get tested if you're unsure
- Vitamin C
- Vitamins A and E
- Vitamin B6 and folate (B9)
- Minerals – zinc, selenium, iron, copper
- Omega-3 fats (EPA/DHA)

If you take a good multivitamin, you'll get your daily dose of vitamin A, E, zinc, iron, copper and selenium, plus B vitamins and others. You'll need to take vitamins D, C and the omega-3 fats as separate supplements. See Part 3 Activate for more on supplements.

As always, please check with your doctor or health practitioner if you are on any medication or have any health conditions.

KEEP YOUR HEART HAPPY

Even though heart disease is often perceived as a 'man's disease', it's the leading cause of death among women over the age of 50. What's even more concerning is that almost two-thirds of women who die suddenly from coronary heart disease show no previous symptoms.

Aside from genetics, going through menopause increases your risk of heart disease. Oestrogen plays a key role in heart health, helping to protect your blood vessels from atherosclerosis, which is the build-up of fatty deposits. So declining levels through menopause can make them more susceptible to damage.

Other significant risk factors for heart disease include high blood pressure, high LDL cholesterol, smoking, lack of exercise, a poor diet, stress, poor sleep, alcohol, insulin resistance, diabetes and obesity.

Blood pressure

High blood pressure or hypertension (over 140/90mmHg) is the most common chronic disease in women over 50, and a significant risk factor for stroke, heart attack, coronary heart disease and kidney disease.

Oestrogen helps blood vessels dilate to ease blood flow, so when levels decline, arteries can narrow and more pressure is needed to get blood through. As well as menopause, other risk factors for high blood pressure include stress, lack of exercise, smoking, obesity, high sodium/low potassium diet, low fibre/high sugar diet, high saturated fat/low omega-3 intakes and diet low in calcium, magnesium and vitamin C.

Cholesterol

If you're postmenopausal, your doctor may have told you that your cholesterol is too high (mine tells me regularly). But unless you have genetically high cholesterol, before you take the recommended cholesterol-lowering medication, please be informed about cholesterol, how it works and its many benefits.

Cholesterol is a good thing. It's a vital building block for the steroid hormones which help control our moods, metabolism, inflammation, immune and sexual functions. The human body needs it in order to function, and without it we would not survive. Cholesterol is also a precursor to vitamin D, another vital hormone.

Focusing solely on lowering your total cholesterol won't necessarily make you less susceptible to heart attacks. There are other critical factors, like inflammation and particle size, that offer a more accurate picture of your heart health risks.

The popular notion that LDL (Low-Density Lipoprotein) is 'bad' cholesterol and HDL (High-Density Lipoprotein) is 'good' cholesterol is an oversimplification of their roles and functions in the body. Both types of lipoproteins serve vital physiological functions, and their 'goodness' or 'badness' is dependent on context, particularly their levels and ratios.

Yet we are still relying on measuring total cholesterol levels and the ratio of LDL to HDL cholesterol to assess a person's risk of developing heart disease. Recent research suggests that measuring the number and size of LDL and HDL particles, and triglyceride levels (blood fats made from sugar) would be a more accurate way to predict risk.

There is even a theory (not proven) that women over 50 make more cholesterol to make up for the lack of steroid hormones as cholesterol converts to 'mother hormone' pregnenolone, which then converts into DHEA, progesterone, testosterone, the oestrogens and cortisol. And it's known that thyroid conditions can have an impact on heart function

It's also important to note that there is a growing concern that treating cholesterol levels too aggressively, such as with medication, can lead to cholesterol levels that are too low. Levels under 4 mmol/l have been shown to potentially increase the risk of dementia in the elderly. For this reason, it's important to work with your healthcare provider to find a treatment plan that balances the benefits of cholesterol-lowering medications with the potential risks of low cholesterol levels.

When evaluating your risk factors, do some critical thinking about what is best for you. If you've been advised to take statin drugs, ask for some hard evidence on why they are recommending them for you. Ask for details of your cholesterol levels, and consider more testing to see if there are other factors that may be at play – jump to Part 3 Beyond Embrace for details.

If your triglycerides are low, your HDL cholesterol optimal (and making up at least one third of your TOTAL cholesterol), chances are you would do better to focus on diet and lifestyle interventions first before starting medication that you'll likely be taking for life.

If you do need to reduce your cholesterol levels, there are some diet and lifestyle protocols that can be very effective.

Dietary advice to reduce saturated fat is well-supported by evidence, though individual responses to fat and dietary cholesterol can vary. However, there's no debate about the need to cut back on sugar, refined carbohydrates, and processed foods. These foods can trigger excess insulin production, prompting the liver to produce more triglycerides—fats that circulate in your bloodstream. Elevated triglyceride levels can disrupt your cholesterol balance, increasing the presence of small, dense LDL particles, which are more likely to contribute to arterial plaque formation than larger, less harmful LDL particles.

Additionally, too much sugar or refined carbs can lower your HDL cholesterol levels (seen to be more protective), creating a lipid profile that's linked to a higher risk of heart disease. Elevated blood sugar can also lead to inflammation, another contributing factor to cardiovascular issues.

It's also vital to manage your stress levels. Just feeling your heart race when you're stressed shows how much it affects us. In the short term, stress triggers hormones like adrenaline and cortisol, which can temporarily increase heart rate and blood pressure. In the long term, chronic stress can lead to persistent high blood pressure, inflammation and changes in heart rhythm, increasing the risk of conditions such as hypertension, heart disease and stroke.

Medication has its place of course (including HRT), but there are many diet and lifestyle interventions that can make a big difference, especially to mild or moderate conditions.

Tips to keep your heart healthy

- **Increase vitamin B3 (niacin):** B3 has been found to raise HDL levels by as much as 24%. The best food sources are liver, chicken, beef, avocados, tomatoes and nuts.

- **Include omega-3s in your diet:** Oily fish, grass-fed beef, free-range organic poultry, nuts, seeds, olives, eggs and avocados are all rich in 'good' fats.
- **Go Mediterranean:** Eating a Mediterranean-style diet with fewer refined carbs, and plenty of vegetables, protein and healthy fats, especially olive oil, can help to lower your triglycerides and raise your HDL.
- **Reduce sodium, increase potassium and magnesium:** Reduce intake of table salt (switch to sea salt which naturally has less sodium), include fresh fruit and vegetables, beans, legumes, nuts and seeds to increase potassium and magnesium.
- **Increase nitric oxide:** This helps vasodilation of our blood vessels, promoting better circulation and blood flow (also helps with sexual function). Eating foods containing nitrates help to increase production, e.g. beetroot, leafy greens, cabbage, celery, rhubarb, parsley. Exposing skin to the sun also triggers nitric oxide.
- **Stop smoking:** Not only does smoking lower your HDL, but it also constricts your blood vessels and raises your risk of heart attack in many other ways as well.
- **Lose weight:** Carrying excess pounds increases your risk of heart disease. Even a little weight reduction can raise your HDL levels.
- **Exercise:** Physical activity not only helps to regulate blood pressure but also raises HDL.
- **Meditation and breathwork:** A recent randomised trial showed that regular meditation decreased the risk of death from heart attack, stroke and all causes by 48%! Nasal breathing is also thought to increase nitric oxide.
- **Prioritise your sleep:** Irregular sleep patterns and duration can double your risk of heart disease so make sure you are doing what you can to improve and regularise your sleep.
- **Helpful supplements:** Multivitamins with active levels of B vitamins, magnesium, potassium, omega-3 DHA/ EPA vitamin D, vitamin K2.

OTHER COMMON SYMPTOMS

Hot or cold? Regulate your body temperature

One of the symptoms that can linger post menopause is difficulty regulating your temperature. If you suffer from hot flushes or night sweats, you'll know how disrupting and unpleasant they can be. It's also common to get cold easily, and at night I'm sure we've all had those duvet off, duvet on nights where you never feel just right!

The decline in oestrogen and progesterone can affect the part of your brain that regulates your body's thermostat, making it harder for you to adjust to different temperatures.

Let's have a look at both extremes.

A hot mess
Hot flushes (or hot flashes) and night sweats are some of the most common symptoms during and post menopause.

One of the biggest benefits of HRT is that it usually deals with hot flushes. However, if it hasn't, or you can't or don't want to take HRT, there are some natural solutions you can try to manage these symptoms.

The first thing to do is be aware of your triggers.

Diet is a big one, with alcohol, caffeine, spicy foods and even food sensitivities like gluten or dairy often being culprits. Stress can be another instigator, and it's not just the external pressures like your job or daily hassles; internal stressors like blood sugar imbalances, dehydration, digestive issues, or nutrient deficiencies can also play a role. These internal factors release cortisol, which can trigger a hot flush.

Smoking is another common cause, and even environmental chemicals and toxins can get you overheated. On top of that, certain medications like antidepressants and hormone treatments can affect your temperature control.

Natural ways to manage hot flushes

- **Avoid your triggers:** Try writing a diary or journal and see whether you can identify any patterns, then try and avoid your specific triggers.
- **Eat phytoestrogens:** Include lots of phytoestrogens, these are plant-based oestrogen-like compounds that can help to regulate your oestrogen levels. Sources include soy (make sure it's organic) and flaxseeds (or linseeds).
- **Manage your stress:** Manage your cortisol through relaxation, lots of self-care, meditation, mindfulness, walks in nature, Epsom salt baths, reading, whatever it is that you do to relax and make sure you're doing it every day for at least 10 to 20 minutes if you can.
- **Minimise your exposure to toxins:** Eat organic as much as possible, filter your tap water, avoid plastics and synthetic fragrances where possible.
- **Regulate your physical body temperature:** Wearing layers, carrying a small fan with you, making sure you're near a window or ventilation, and using natural fabrics for your clothes and bedding can all be helpful in minimising discomfort.
- **Supplements:** Try taking my recommended supplements for your basic nutrients (see Part 3), then if you're not taking HRT, you can add in a formula that includes some phytoestrogens (such as red clover, sage, hops) which can be very helpful.

Always cold

As well as your body feeling hot, many women report feeling colder than usual too. It could be that your metabolism is slowing down, and you're naturally generating less internal heat than before. Additionally, your blood vessels lose some of their elasticity, and this can lead to less efficient circulation, particularly in the extremities.

Another important thing to check is your thyroid (we covered this in Part 1). Low thyroid function, also known as hypothyroidism, can make you more sensitive to cold temperatures. The thyroid gland plays a vital role in regulating your metabolism, which includes your body's ability to produce heat. When your thyroid hormones are too low, your metabolic rate can drop, making it more difficult for your body to generate adequate heat.

Keeping yourself warm is really important, not only for your own comfort but for your body to function properly. Wearing several layers of clothing can trap warm air close to your body. Opt for thermal or moisture-wicking base layers and top with a warm sweater and coat. Always keep your feet, hands and head well-insulated, as these areas lose heat quickly.

Movement can help increase your core body temperature. Even a brief walk can get your blood flowing and help you feel warmer. Consider using hot water bottles, heat pads or electric blankets to provide external sources of warmth. And ensure your environment is well-insulated and heated.

It's especially important to get your thyroid tested to make sure you're not deficient (more on this in Part 3).

Skin, hair and nail health – finding your glow

As we navigate life after menopause, changes to our skin, hair and nails are inevitable. Yet, they are closely tied to our overall wellbeing and can even offer clues about what's happening beneath the surface.

Skin health

One of the first things you might notice about getting older is how your skin changes. Oestrogen makes skin plump and supple. It has a significant role in collagen production, which provides structure and elasticity to tissues such as skin, bones and joints. So, when oestrogen levels decline, you may notice an increase in wrinkles, a decrease in elasticity, more pigmentation or 'age spots'. These changes can be further exacerbated by exposure to environmental factors like the sun and pollution.

Conditions like rosacea, characterised by facial redness and small bumps, often become more noticeable. Adult acne may also occur due to hormonal fluctuations. Eczema and psoriasis can either emerge or worsen too.

Skin appearance is something that matters a lot to most women, so these changes can be tough to handle. After all, that's why the cosmetic surgery industry is thriving!

So firstly, let's take a moment to revisit the Positive Ageing section in Part 1. Reframing your attitude towards how you look is an important step towards acceptance and finding peace with it.

Secondly, your skin is a mirror to your inner health. Issues may be 'managed' by topical creams or aesthetic treatments, but your diet and lifestyle can have a huge impact from the inside out.

For starters, hydration is key; not just topically but also internally. Drinking enough water can help keep your skin plump and minimise the appearance of wrinkles.

In terms of your diet, antioxidants are your skin's best friends – think berries, colourful veggies, nuts and seeds. They can help fight free radical damage. Omega-3 fatty acids found in fish like salmon can also improve skin elasticity. Incorporating foods high in vitamins A, C and E can further boost your skin's health.

In terms of lifestyle, regular exercise can improve your circulation, nourishing your skin and keeping it vibrant. Sleep is another helper, revitalising your skin as much as any topical treatment.

While topical skin treatments can be beneficial – look for ingredients like retinol, hyaluronic acid or vitamin C – make sure your products are as natural as possible. Your skin absorbs everything you put on it, directly into the bloodstream. Be mindful of products that contain parabens, phthalates, fragrance, parfum and other chemicals. You don't want to take on more toxins than necessary.

Sunscreen is also vital. It protects against both UVA and UVB rays that can exacerbate signs of ageing and increase your risk of skin cancer. Unfortunately many mainstream suncare brands contain toxic ingredients that can not only mess with your hormones, but ironically can also cause cancer – the very thing you're trying to protect yourself from! (More on this in Part 3 Eliminate.)

Taking a holistic approach that combines natural skincare with a balanced diet and a healthy lifestyle can go a long way in maintaining good skin health as you age. And acknowledging that your skin won't look the same as it did when you were younger, will help you feel more positive about getting older.

Hair
Post menopause, many women experience changes in their hair. It can become thinner, drier and more prone to breakage. You may notice a shift in the texture of your hair, as it becomes coarser or frizzier.

One of the most distressing changes for many women is hair loss. While it's often associated with ageing in men, it's a surprisingly common symptom among women as well. Since many women link their hair to feelings of attractiveness, experiencing hair loss can be really upsetting.

Female hair loss can have multiple triggers, each with its own underlying causes and potential solutions.

Stress, both physical and emotional, can temporarily hinder hair growth as the body prioritises essential functions during survival mode.

Thyroid issues, common among women over 40, can also impact hair health due to their role in cellular energy supply.

Autoimmune alopecia, where the immune system targets hair follicles, often stems from gut issues and demands professional investigation.

Genetic predisposition, menopausal hormone fluctuations and high levels of testosterone or its potent form, DHT, can further contribute to hair thinning. Conditions like PCOS and rapid weight loss amplify the issue, as do certain medications such as birth control, NSAIDs like ibuprofen, and antidepressants. You may want to discuss possible side effects with your doctor.

Check your hair products and styling routine – make sure your products are toxin-free and don't overstyle your hair. Be careful of colouring too – chemicals from colour products can be very damaging – and go for more natural brands or visit an organic salon.

And lastly make sure you're including these nutrients in your diet or supplement routine: iron, biotin, zinc, collagen, silica, choline, B vitamins, vitamin D, protein, and omega-3 fats.

Nails
Another important concern to many women is their nails. They might start growing slower or becoming more brittle and prone to breakage. They can also lose some of their natural shine and moisture, feeling drier and rougher to the touch. Sometimes, you might even see ridges or discoloration on the nail surface. These changes are normal as we age and are often influenced by factors like hormonal shifts and overall health.

Taking good care of your nails, keeping them moisturised and avoiding harsh chemicals, can help keep them looking their best as you age. Additionally, ensuring you get enough nutrients like biotin, vitamin E, iron, zinc and protein in your diet can support nail health and strength.

Do watch out for the type of nail polish and nail polish removers you're using as many contain toxic chemicals such as formaldehyde, toluene, dibutyl phthalate, camphor and harsh solvents which can pose health risks including irritation, allergic reactions and long-term health effects. There are many natural alternatives available.

Migraines: find the root cause

According to research undertaken in 2003, it is estimated that there are 190,000 migraine attacks experienced every day in England! Six million people suffer from migraines in the UK, with women much more susceptible than men.

For women, migraines can have a few different causal factors.

Hormonal shifts, particularly decreases in oestrogen and progesterone during menstruation or menopause, are recognised triggers. Additionally, inadequate serotonin levels play a significant role in pain regulation, influenced by factors such as low oestrogen, insufficient sunlight exposure and deficiencies in nutrients like vitamin B6, C, magnesium, and zinc.

Poor gut health can also impact serotonin production. And inflammation in the gut (caused by microbial imbalances or food sensitivities) can directly increase inflammation in the brain, which can then trigger migraines.

Stress, whether emotional or physical, can alter neuro-transmitter function and increase tension, triggering migraines. Even sleep patterns matter – too little, too much, or irregular sleep can set the stage for a migraine episode.

Other contributing factors include certain medications, systemic inflammation, hormone-disrupting chemicals and musculoskeletal factors, such as injury or inflammation in muscles or ligaments.

Natural approaches to migraines

- **Know your triggers:** keep a diary so you know what might trigger them and avoid your triggers as much as possible.
- **Eat anti-inflammatory foods:** lots of antioxidants (fruit and veg), herbs, spices, healthy fats.
- **Avoid inflammatory foods:** including sugar, refined carbs, bad fats (veg oils), processed foods, alcohol.
- **Avoid food sensitivities** (e.g. gluten, dairy) for three to four weeks and note any symptom changes.
- **Eat omega-3 fats** from oily fish (or take a supplement) to fight inflammation and support your brain cell health.
- **Keep blood sugar stable** to balance insulin and cortisol.
- **Liver support:** support your liver with cruciferous vegetables and a liver supplement formula (including milk thistle).
- **Include phytoestrogens** in your diet (if you're menopausal and not taking HRT) such as organic soy, flaxseeds, chickpeas and lentils.
- **Support your gut:** eat lots of prebiotic and probiotic foods.
- **Keep hydrated** and avoid caffeine if it's a trigger.
- **Manage stress:** meditation and breathwork or jump to Rest in Part 3.
- **Supplements:** take my basic top five (see Activate in Part 3), and studies suggest riboflavin at 400mg can also help (check with your doctor if you're on any medication).
- **Get yourself tested** to rule out any hormone imbalances, gut issues or nutrient deficiencies.

PART 3

EMBRACE:

Your Healthy Ageing Toolkit

We've looked at specific areas of the body and mind that might need some immediate help, but now let's focus on putting your health jigsaw puzzle together so that you can stay as healthy as possible as you get older.

I fully intend to EMBRACE the next chapter of my life and to do that I need to be physically and mentally healthy and functional. So, I have put together all my clinical experience, knowledge and research into my EMBRACE protocol.

I have designed this protocol to support your physical and mental health as you enter the next chapter of your life. It's designed to switch on your longevity genes and protective anti-ageing pathways and turn down your inflammatory and pro-ageing pathways.

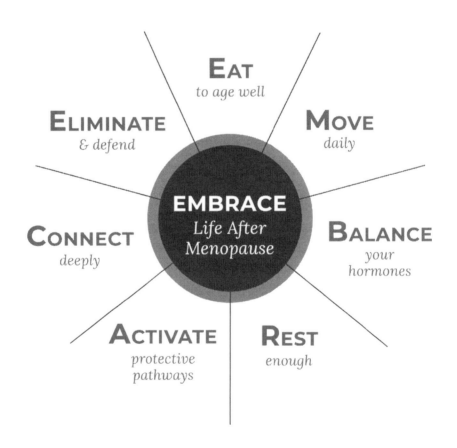

Some of it will feel familiar if you've read my previous book and come across my four-step 'Happy Hormone Code' but this protocol goes much further than just balancing your hormones. It's a guide to looking after your whole body and mind as you enter this next chapter.

Again, please don't feel that you have to do it all! Take the bits that work for you and maybe try a few new things if they feel appropriate. What counts isn't any one action we take, but the consistent daily habits we cultivate.

Don't forget to download your free workbook to complete yourself at: www.happyhormonesforlife.com/life

CHAPTER 6

E – EAT to age well

I have to start with what's on your plate. Why? Because the food you consume doesn't just fill you up; it fundamentally influences how you feel today and how well you'll age in the future.

Hippocrates famously said, "Let food be thy medicine", but food can also be thy poison!

Your 50 trillion (or so) cells rely on nutrients to run your body. If any of those nutrients are missing, your cells aren't going to have what they need to function optimally, and that's going to potentially impact your health now and in the future.

What's more, we know that our nutritional needs increase as we get older due to several factors:

- Our metabolism slows down, leading to less efficient nutrient absorption.
- Our muscle mass decreases, requiring more protein to maintain strength and function.
- Our bone density reduces, necessitating higher intake of calcium and vitamin D.
- Our immune system weakens, making antioxidants and essential vitamins more critical for maintaining overall health and preventing chronic diseases.

Additionally, age-related health conditions and medications can affect nutrient requirements and absorption.

A study done in 2024 showed that postmenopausal women are

at increased risk of nutrient imbalances, including lower levels of omega-3s, vitamin D and B vitamins, along with higher levels of iron, which may predispose them to certain chronic diseases.

This just makes it extra important that we make sure our diet is the best it can be, and that we're supplementing the right nutrients (more on that under Activate).

Your diet is a powerful tool that can either activate or silence your genes, which can shape your susceptibility to chronic disease.

The great thing is that YOU control what, when and how you eat. Every day, your food choices and dietary patterns serve as a daily prescription for your long-term wellbeing.

But how exactly do you make the right choices? You wouldn't be alone if you're scratching your head about this. We're bombarded with messages about which diets are the best ones to follow, whether it's keto, paleo, pescatarian, carnivore, vegan, low carb, low calorie, high fat, high protein, the list goes on …

The truth is there is no miracle one diet for everyone. You have to experiment and find out what works for your unique body. But there are some general principles that do work for most of us.

I've mentioned the Blue Zone centenarians, and while their diets differ variably, there are similarities that unite them. Only one region is totally vegan, but they all eat lots of REAL FOOD: fresh vegetables, fruits, legumes, nuts and whole grains. They all include sources of healthy fats, such as olive oil in Mediterranean Blue Zones and nuts in others. Even alcohol is not a total no-no, as Greece and Sardinia include locally produced wine in their diets (but only drink in moderation and socially). And not surprisingly, there's very few (if any) processed or sugary foods consumed.

One thing they don't do is count calories. They naturally eat what they need, many of them eating until they are almost full.

The first step in crafting your healthy ageing eating strategy involves distinguishing between foods that nourish us as we age and those that accelerate the ageing process.

AGEING FOODS

Let's dive into the foods that we need to be looking at reducing.

Sugar

We now know how damaging sugar can be to our health and longevity. Remember the section on 'glycation' or 'death by sugar'? This is when glucose molecules can attach themselves to proteins and cause damage or stop them working at all. This creates AGE products (Advanced Glycation End), and the more they accumulate the faster we age.

However, even though we know about the dangers of sugar, for many of us it's really hard to live a sugar-free lifestyle. David Gillespie, author of *Sweet Poison*, states: "Very few of us are making conscious decisions about the sugar we eat. The average Briton is consuming more than a kilo – 238 teaspoonfuls – a week, but I bet they'd be flummoxed accounting for more than a few teaspoons of that. Sugar is deeply and thoroughly embedded in our food supply."

Let's dig into where sugar is lurking. There are three main types to be aware of:

1. Refined sugar you might add to drinks (e.g. tea, coffee) or when baking.
2. Hidden sugars in processed foods and drinks – look for sugar in the ingredients list in sauces, dressings, cereals, ready meals, fruit juices, soft drinks, etc. It can be disguised as syrups, juices or anything ending in -ose.
3. Natural sugars in fruit, honey, dried fruits, alcohol.

Reducing sugar that you're adding to your food or drink is obviously the first (and easiest) thing to do. Next is recognising the hidden sugar in processed foods (and drinks) that many of us consume unconsciously.

This hidden sugar can rack up on a daily basis when you are eating ready meals, baked goods, fruit yoghurts, cereal bars, sauces, fruit smoothies, juices and many low-fat products – these are the things that account for most of our sugar intake. Start reading labels. If sugar or one of its many guises is listed in the first three ingredients, you really want to be avoiding it.

If you reduce refined and hidden sugars, you can then enjoy the sugar that is derived from natural sources – in moderation and as long as it hasn't been too processed (for instance, choose raw honey over processed honey, fresh fruit over fruit juice). Sugar is sugar after all, but at least natural foods usually come with fibre and other nutrients that help the body process the sugars.

And don't be tempted to swap to DIET (or No Added Sugar) products – these contain artificial sweeteners that can potentially interfere with metabolic processes and contribute to weight gain, metabolic syndrome and increased risk of chronic disease.

The good news is that as you reduce your sugar intake, you'll retrain your taste buds. Not only will your cravings diminish, but food will also start tasting sweeter, making you realise you need less sugar than before.

Refined carbohydrates

We all know sugar when we see it, so we can choose to have it or not. What we don't often realise is that ALL carbohydrates are essentially long chains of sugar molecules strung together with various structural complexities.

And when we eat carbs, whether it's white bread or a plate of healthy vegetables, our digestive system breaks that down into simple sugars like glucose, which enter the bloodstream.

That process is totally normal, it's how our cells get the energy they need. The problem comes with the type of carbs we're eating.

Not all carbs have the same impact on the body. With refined or 'simple' carbs such as most bread, cereals, pastries, pasta and pre-packaged snacks, the sugar is very quickly broken down and absorbed, leading to quick spikes in blood sugar and insulin levels. These are classified as high glycaemic index (or load) foods.

However, the sugar found in complex carbs, such as vegetables, whole grains and legumes is broken down much more slowly. This is because the sugar molecules are arranged in more complex structures and often accompanied by fibre, vitamins and minerals, which slow the whole process down, reducing the impact on your blood sugar. These are classified as low glycaemic index (or load) foods.

That's why it's important to 'put some clothes on your carbs' as advised by Jessie Inchauspé, otherwise known as the 'Glucose Goddess'. Never let your carbs go naked, which essentially means add protein or fat to your carbs to reduce the blood sugar spike. For me, that looks like adding avocado and smoked salmon to my piece of toast (also choosing good bread like sourdough or seeded). Or having an apple with a piece of cheese, some nuts or nut butter.

Other tricks to reduce the impact of carbs include eating your veggies first, so that the fibre can take hold and slow down the sugar breakdown. Walking after a meal can also help limit a blood sugar spike, as can taking a sip of vinegar before a meal (I like apple cider vinegar with the 'mother' in it for a microbiome boost).

Alcohol
While locally grown organic wine does feature in a couple of the Blue Zones, alcohol in general is not your ageing friend.

It's no secret that I'm a wine and gin lover, so when I look at the evidence on alcohol and ageing, it really isn't my favourite research! But I'm also painfully aware of the negative effects of alcohol on my body these days, so I'm naturally drinking much less. And I know I'm not alone in this, I see similar behaviour in midlife women around me.

If you're needing some motivation to drink less, read on.

Weight gain: It's a bit more complex than just the 'empty' calories, alcohol messes with your blood sugar – and we know what the consequences of that are by now!

Mood and stress: After the initial happy feelings, alcohol can lower serotonin levels, leaving you prone to low mood and depression. The thing many women use it for – to de-stress – is actually raising your stress hormone cortisol, making you more anxious and overwhelmed in the long run. It can also lower testosterone, affecting your libido, motivation and sense of wellbeing.

Brain health: That hangover isn't just an uncomfortable aftermath of a good night. It's been shown that just one glass of wine (or other unit) a day can damage neurons and cells in the brain, increasing inflammation and risk of dementia. And I'm afraid it's even more toxic in women than men due to our hormones, liver and biochemistry.

Sleep: Alcohol can help you fall asleep initially, but having an evening drink can reduce your deep sleep and wake you up at 3am with low blood sugar and/or dehydration – both of which are stresses on the body, raising cortisol.

Your liver: Your liver is already struggling – with all the toxins we have around, plus the hormones that we need to detoxify. Alcohol produces acetaldehyde which if not detoxified quickly can result in headaches, nausea, brain fog and fatigue – a typical 'hangover'.

Your gut: Alcohol can damage the cells in the lining of your gut, increasing inflammation and the risk of leaky gut which can lead to autoimmune conditions. Alcohol can also alter nutrient absorption as it can reduce enzyme production for digesting food.

Nutritional deficiencies: Alcohol's diuretic properties can result in the leaching of vital vitamins and minerals from the body, including antioxidants like vitamins A and C that are essential for cell repair and regeneration. Over time, this can result in prematurely aged skin and a decrease in the body's overall ability to repair itself.

Bone health: We know that alcohol leads to bone loss, as it inhibits osteoblasts – your bone building cells, alters vitamin D, testosterone and cortisol – which all impact bone health.

Longevity: No surprise, alcohol doesn't help you live longer! Evidence shows it leads to more strokes, fatal aneurysms, heart failure and mortality. In the UK, alcohol is one of the top five causes of death and disability, and the most common cause of death in men under 50.

If you have decided to break up with alcohol, I applaud you! I've no doubt your health will be better for it. But if you're not quite able to give up completely, the good news is that even small reductions in alcohol use can make a big difference. Professor David Nutt, leading researcher in alcohol use, advises women to consume no more than 15g of alcohol per day (roughly equivalent to a glass of wine) and to have at least two alcohol-free days per week.

Here are some more tips for managing alcohol:

- **Always have food** if you're drinking alcohol – never drink on an empty stomach.
- **Choose wine over cocktails or spirits** with sugary mixer (and don't do diet mixers) – red wine is best as you tend to drink less, and it's got some antioxidants (although watchout if you're histamine intolerant).
- **Start swapping in zero-alcohol alternatives** to see if it's the ritual rather than the drink that you're craving. There are some great brands available now, or you can try a kombucha, coconut water or sparkling water with lemon/lime. Pour into a wine glass if that helps.
- **Always stay hydrated** – drink water before, during, in between and after alcohol.
- **Have 'alcohol free' days** – as many as possible.
- **Take a longer break** as often as possible – e.g. dry January or join a club to help you give up forever.
- **Choose quality** over quantity.
- Ask yourself if it's just a habit, or you really WANT it.
- **Don't drink at night if you don't sleep well** or if you suffer hangovers the next day.
- **Alcohol cravings** can happen when your blood sugar is low – mine happen just as I'm starting to cook dinner! Try a large glass of water with a handful of nuts – the craving should pass.
- **Eat lots of cruciferous vegetable**s (broccoli, cauliflower, cabbage, kale, chard, rocket, Brussels sprouts, watercress, etc.) – to help your liver detox your oestrogen.
- **Take a good multivitamin** with good levels of active B vitamins (including folate) – plus a liver formula with milk thistle, N-Acetyl Cysteine and other liver helpers (see Part 3 Eliminate).

Vegetable oils

Eating vegetable and plant oils (e.g. vegetable, sunflower, corn, soy, rapeseed, canola) can speed up ageing because they're mainly made up of omega-6 fatty acids, which can cause inflammation and oxidative stress when not balanced with omega-3s. These oils are fairly cheap, so tend to be used in processing, such as refining, heating, bleaching and deodorising, which can create harmful compounds like advanced glycation end products (AGEs) and trans fats, both of which can contribute to ageing by promoting inflammation and damaging cells.

Vegetable oils are also used in anything that is deep fried, including chips, fried chicken, donuts, battered foods, tempura vegetables, onion rings, hash browns, mozzarella sticks, etc.

Minimise processed foods (see next section) and fried foods, and stick to olive oil and stable fats like butter, lard and coconut oil for cooking. Use small amounts of other cold pressed oils for drizzling and flavour.

Processed foods

We all know the obvious drawbacks of processed foods (particularly ultra-processed foods), but what's even more alarming for us as we age is their role in promoting inflammation.

The combination of sugar, salt, vegetable oils, additives and preservatives are a recipe for inflammation. On top of that, these foods often lack essential nutrients like antioxidants, fibre and healthy fats that fight inflammation. A double whammy.

Not all processed foods are bad though, which is why I tend to focus on 'ultra' processed foods as the ones to really avoid.

Some ultra-processed foods to minimise:

- Ready meals, sauces, salad dressings, instant soups and gravy
- Fast food, takeaways
- Breakfast cereals
- Mass-produced bread (white and brown)
- Processed meats (low-quality bacon, sausages, burgers, etc.)
- Margarine and spreads
- Processed cheeses (slices, strings, etc.)
- Crisps, popcorn and savoury snacks (including vegetable crisps)
- Cookies, pastries, cakes, biscuits, chocolate, confectionery, sweet snacks
- Ice cream and ready-made desserts
- Fizzy drinks, energy drinks, fruit juices and smoothies
- Vegan fake meats, cheeses

Check your labels, choose brands that use olive oil or avocado over vegetable oils, reduced (or no) sugar, and generally ingredients that you recognise.

Healthier processed foods: You don't need to sacrifice convenience completely. Here are some healthier processed foods that I regularly buy; cooked quinoa, tinned fish, cans or jars of chickpeas, beans, pulses, organic tomato pasta sauces, jars of artichokes or peppers, nut butters, frozen fruit/veg, pesto, oatcakes, good quality mayonnaise, tahini and low-sugar granolas.

Food sensitivities

If you're sensitive to certain foods, it can not only cause discomfort or painful symptoms, but can contribute to inflammation and faster ageing. However, we must distinguish between food *allergies* and food *intolerances* or *sensitivities*. The former can kill you (or seriously harm you), the latter can result in mildly or seriously uncomfortable symptoms. And in my experience, food sensitivities can be a sign that your gut isn't happy, but by improving your gut health, you might be able to eliminate them entirely.

- LIFE AFTER MENOPAUSE -

Common intolerances include gluten, dairy, soy, grains, eggs, corn, nuts, nightshades and certain fruit or vegetables. Gluten and dairy are the most common, but do watch out for alternatives. The 'free from' industry has grown into a huge beast. While choice is great, many of these products are highly processed and use additives, oils and sugar to produce them. Read labels carefully, and either steer clear or make your own 'free from' alternatives.

Gluten

Gluten refers to a group of proteins found in grains such as wheat, rye, barley and spelt. The main proteins in it are gliadin and glutenin, with gliadin mostly responsible for the negative effects. There are three main conditions that are medically recognised:

- **Coeliac disease:** About 1% of the population have been diagnosed (many more are likely to be undiagnosed) with coeliac disease, which is an autoimmune reaction to gluten that damages the gut's villi, leading to digestive issues, nutrient deficiencies, anaemia and a higher risk of other autoimmune diseases.
- **Non-coeliac gluten sensitivity** (NCGS) is the most common and often unrecognised form of gluten-related disorder. While coeliac disease represents the 'end stage' of gluten sensitivity, NCGS encompasses a range of issues caused by gluten without necessarily progressing to coeliac disease. NCGS is now a recognised medical condition for individuals who test negative for coeliac disease.
- **Wheat allergy** is an immune response, not autoimmune, involving IgE antibodies that attack wheat proteins. You may be allergic to wheat but tolerate other grains. It's also possible to have both a wheat allergy and gluten sensitivity.

Symptoms of gluten sensitivity or intolerance can cause digestive issues such as IBS, diarrhoea, constipation, bloating, gas, pain. But other symptoms unrelated to the gut can include fatigue, brain fog, headaches, hormonal issues, weight gain, mood issues, joint pain, skin issues and more. In fact, because it can cause inflammation, symptoms can show up pretty much anywhere in the body.

The key underlying factors in gluten sensitivity are genetics (determined by the HLA gene), dysbiosis (microbiome imbalance) and leaky gut, where gluten causes inflammation and holes in the gut wall.

If you suspect you have an issue with gluten, you should get tested for coeliac disease and wheat allergy first and foremost. If these are negative, it doesn't rule out a gluten sensitivity. However, there is no standard medical test for gluten sensitivity, and many of the intolerance testing on the market can be unreliable. The best way to find out is to remove gluten-containing foods (and drinks) from your diet for a minimum of 30 days, then re-introduce them. If symptoms improve during elimination then return on re-introduction, your body is telling you something!

Dairy

I'll come to whether dairy is 'healthy' or not in the next section, but it's going to be something you want to avoid if you have an intolerance to it.

There are two main types of dairy intolerance:

- **Lactose intolerance:** This isn't actually an intolerance as such, it's due to a deficiency in the enzyme lactase, which is needed to digest lactose, the sugar found in dairy products. Without enough lactase, lactose remains undigested in the gut, leading to symptoms such as bloating, gas, diarrhoea, pain and discomfort. Lactose intolerance is often genetic and more prevalent in certain populations, particularly those of Asian, African and Native American descent, and tends to increase with age.
- **Dairy protein allergies:** This is an immune reaction to proteins found in dairy products, such as casein and

whey. Symptoms can range from mild to severe and may include skin rashes, hives, swelling, digestive issues, respiratory problems and even anaphylaxis in rare cases. Unlike lactose intolerance, which is a problem with digestion, dairy protein allergies involve an immune response to specific proteins in dairy products.

While lactose intolerance may require avoiding or reducing lactose-containing foods or using lactase supplements, dairy protein allergies typically necessitate complete avoidance of dairy products.

If you have symptoms that are unresolved, you may want to try an elimination diet and remove dairy from your diet for 30 days, then reintroduce products one at a time, starting with sheep or goats cheese, butter, cream, cows cheese, yoghurt and lastly milk. Leave two days between each re-introduction to notice any symptoms.

Another option if you're reacting to milk is to switch to A2 cows milk. A1 milk, from modern cow breeds like Holsteins, contains A1 beta-casein protein which can cause digestive issues, while A2 milk, from traditional breeds like Jerseys and Guernseys, contains only A2 beta-casein, which is easier to digest.

HEALTHY AGEING FOODS

The good news is that there are SO many great foods to choose from that are going to help us age well.

Let's go through the ones you need to focus on.

Macronutrients

Macronutrients are the building blocks of our diet, and each one plays a unique role in our health, from fuelling our cells and supporting our brain function to keeping our hormones in check.

PROTEIN

If you're navigating midlife or beyond, chances are you're not getting enough protein. And that's a bigger deal than you might think. As levels of oestrogen and progesterone drop, we need to eat more protein in our diet because our bodies are less efficient at absorbing and using it properly.

Protein, the essential building block of life, is vital for tissue growth, repair and maintenance in our bodies. It helps develop muscles and organs, strengthens bones, supports cell signalling, and is involved in many other crucial processes that help us age well:

Muscle preservation and strength: Protein helps counteract muscle loss by providing the amino acids needed to preserve and build lean muscle tissue.

Weight management: Protein is a big helper for midlife weight gain. Here's why:

- It has a high satiety value, meaning it keeps you feeling fuller for longer. This can help regulate appetite and prevent overeating.
- It can boost your metabolism. It has a higher thermic effect compared to carbohydrates and fats, meaning it requires more energy to digest and metabolise. This can result in more calories being burnt.
- It can help regulate your appetite by reducing ghrelin (your hunger hormone) and increasing peptide YY (PYY), a hormone that makes you feel full.

Protein can also change your shape. A recent study of overweight women found that those who ate a high protein diet (1.8g of protein per kg of body weight), dropped from 35% body fat to 20% body fat after 12 weeks compared to the control group.

Blood sugar regulation: Protein-rich foods help to slow down the absorption of glucose into the bloodstream, preventing spikes and crashes in blood sugar.

Insulin sensitivity: Protein consumption can enhance insulin sensitivity, which helps to promote hormone balance and reduces the risk of inflammation, insulin resistance and metabolic disorders.

Bone health: It's a common misconception that only calcium and vitamin D matter when it comes to your bones – actually protein makes up a significant part of bone composition. This is especially crucial for postmenopausal women who are at a higher risk for osteoporosis.

Heart health: Consuming adequate protein, particularly from sources such as poultry, fish, legumes and nuts, can help regulate blood pressure levels, increase nitric oxide, and help to improve cholesterol profile.

Mental wellbeing: Amino acids support the production of neurotransmitters, including serotonin, which plays a crucial role in mood regulation.

Immune system: Protein helps produce antibodies, enzymes and immune system cells, strengthening the body's defences and reducing the risk of infections and illness.

There's a huge amount of debate (and therefore confusion!) about how much protein we need to eat. And it also varies based on factors such as individual health, activity level, stage of life and muscle mass.

A key amino acid called leucine (one of the branched-chain amino acids) helps to stimulate mTOR activity. mTOR is one of the nutrient signalling pathways we covered in Chapter 3, a protein that helps regulate cell growth, cell proliferation, muscle synthesis and cell survival. But it only works over a certain amount, commonly called the 'leucine threshold'. As we age, it's harder for us to reach this threshold, which is why we need to include more protein in our diet.

In a bid to cut through some of the confusion, experts in

nutrition for older people got together to form the PROT-AGE Study Group, where they conducted research on protein needs and lifestyle approaches for maintaining muscle in older age. They recommend a daily protein intake of 1.0 to 1.2g per kilogram of body weight for healthy older adults, however if you exercise, this rises to 1.5-2g per kg of body weight.

That means if you weigh 70kg and are healthy, your base target would be 70–83g per day, but with exercise it's 105–140g per day. That's 30–50g per meal. Now this is a lot more than the NHS recommended amount of 0.75g/kg of body weight, however unless you have kidney or other health conditions, studies show that it's a good target for most.

The type of protein is also important. Animal proteins are considered complete sources of protein, containing all essential amino acids in the right proportions, while most plant proteins lack one or more essential amino acids, making them incomplete sources. So, if you're a vegetarian or vegan, you need to make sure you're eating a wide variety of protein sources and combining them to provide a balanced amino acid profile. Common examples are rice and beans, hummus and wholegrain bread, tofu and rice, lentils and barley, peanut butter with wholegrain toast.

I will always recommend you get your protein from food, but a good-quality protein powder can offer a convenient, quick and reliable source, ensuring that even on hectic days, you can meet your dietary protein requirements and support healthy ageing. A quick green protein smoothie for breakfast is a great way to set you up for the day. Look for high-quality protein sources (e.g. organic whey, pea, hemp), minimal additives, low sugar content, third-party testing for purity, a balanced nutritional profile, allergen-free options and good digestibility.

Typical protein content in some common foods

If you're wondering how much protein you're consuming and looking for easy ways to increase it, here are some approximate values for some common foods:

- 1 egg (medium) – 7g
- 1 tbsp peanut butter – 7g
- 1 cup tofu – 30g
- Chicken breast – 30g
- Salmon fillet – 30g
- Tin of tuna – 22g
- Handful of almonds – 6g
- 1 cup of quinoa – 16g
- ½ small tub of cottage cheese (150g) – 16g
- 1 cup broccoli – 2.5g
- 1/2 cup of chickpeas – 8g
- 1 cup of lentils – 18g
- 1 cup of pinto beans – 15g
- Pot of plain soy yoghurt (150g) – 9g
- Pot of Greek yoghurt (150g) – 14g
- 400ml glass of whole milk – 14g
- 500ml glass of kefir milk – 9g
- 100g of parmesan cheese – 35g
- 1 medium slice of sourdough bread – 8g
- 1 tbsp nutritional yeast flakes – 4g
- 1 tbsp chia seeds – 3g
- ½ avocado – 1.5g
- Whey or plant protein shake – approx. 30g (you may need to supplement plant protein powder with branched-chain amino acids, leucine or creatine)

Here are some ideas for a protein-rich breakfast to kickstart your day (each should come to around 20–30g):

- 2 eggs with 2 pieces free-range bacon or smoked salmon, half avocado on sourdough toast.
- 3-egg omelette with cheese, ham, broccoli, sprinkling of pumpkin/sunflower seeds
- Greek yoghurt with berries, nuts and seeds (or home-made granola), slice of sourdough toast with nut butter.
- Tofu scramble – mash or grate your tofu, then fry with olive oil, spring onions, garlic, spices of choice. Add a tbsp of nutritional yeast flakes, beans or cottage cheese for an extra taste and protein hit.
- Protein smoothie with plant or whey protein powder, nut butter, flax and chia seeds

Add in your veg wherever possible – spinach, kale, cabbage, broccoli, mushrooms, tomatoes – all great options to add in with eggs.

Remember, quality matters! Opt for complete proteins like grass-fed red meat, fish, poultry, eggs, and plant-based options like legumes, tofu and quinoa, organic where possible.

FAT
For years, we've been advised to avoid fat because it was believed to cause obesity and heart disease. This guidance stems from research conducted in the 1950s, which continues to influence health policy and medical opinions today, despite having been debunked by modern scientists.

The tragedy is that this low-fat policy has harmed us by encouraging us to avoid fats that are actually essential for our wellbeing and play a significant role in the ageing process. And studies have shown that it has likely encouraged increased consumption of sugar and carbohydrates, contributing to the current obesity and health epidemic.

Here are some of the many benefits of healthy fats:

- **Brain health:** Your brain is made up of 60% fat – keeping your brain healthy is key to ageing well.
- **Cellular health:** Every cell in your body needs fat for the membranes to work properly.
- **Blood sugar:** Fat helps to fill you up and prevent those between meal sugar/carb cravings – balancing your blood sugar and insulin production.
- **Vitamin absorption:** Fat helps you absorb your fat-soluble vitamins (A, D, E,K) – helping your hormones to work properly.
- **Immune support:** Healthy fats help to reduce inflammation and support your immune system.
- **Heart health:** Fats help to support your cardiovascular system and healthy cholesterol (see more on cholesterol and how to improve your heart health in Part 2: Keep Your Heart Happy).
- **Skin and bone health:** Fats help to keep your skin supple and bones strong.
- **And weight loss?** It's actually low-carb not low-fat diets that have consistently performed better for weight loss in the general population.

Unfortunately, it's not as simple as saying fats are 'good' or 'bad'. Dietary fats are divided into three main groups:

- Saturated fatty acids (SAFAs) – short, medium and long chain
- Mono-unsaturated fatty acids (MUFAs) – medium and long chain
- Poly-unsaturated fatty acids (PUFAs) – long chain

For years, we've been advised to avoid saturated fats and consume more monounsaturated and polyunsaturated fats. However, all foods that naturally contain fat have a mixture of different types of fats. You can't separate foods by fat type since they all contain a bit of everything.

This is why it's misleading to say, 'Don't eat red meat – it's full of saturated fat'. Red meat also contains PUFAs and MUFAs! Nature combines various fats in foods for a reason, as our bodies utilise them for different purposes.

The secret is to eat as many real, natural, minimally processed foods as possible, and focus on 'healthy' fat-containing foods such as grass-fed meat, free-range poultry, oily fish, organic full-fat dairy, eggs, nuts, seeds, avocadoes, olives, cold pressed seed/nut oils.

The 'essential' fats
While the body can synthesise most of the fats it requires, omega-3 and omega-6 fatty acids are exceptions, known as 'essential fats', because they must be obtained from dietary sources or supplements. It's vital to consume adequate amounts of these fats and maintain the correct balance between them.

However, omega-6 fatty acids are readily available in modern diets, primarily from sources like vegetable oils and animal products, while omega-3 fatty acids, found in oily fish, nuts and seeds, are less prevalent. As a result, the ratio of omega-6 to omega-3 fats has increased, corresponding with the rise in consumption of margarine and processed foods, alongside the decline in oily fish intake.

Patrick Holford claims in his book *Upgrade Your Brain* that the decline in omega-3 fats coupled with increased consumption of sugary, processed foods is a significant factor contributing to shrinking brain sizes and declining IQ rates since the 1970s. This trend coincided with the demonisation of dietary fats and the rise in popularity of high-sugar processed foods.

The three main omega-3 fatty acids are alpha-linolenic acid (ALA), eicosapentaenoic acid (EPA), and docosahexaenoic acid (DHA). These fatty acids play crucial roles in various bodily functions, particularly DHA which is essential for the brain, eyes and nervous system, and EPA which is anti-inflammatory and aids heart health.

DHA and EPA are only found in fatty fish or algae. ALA is found in flaxseeds, chia seeds and walnuts, however ALA needs to go through a complex conversion process to get to the EPA and DHA omega-3 fats that the body can use. So, if you're plant-based or not eating oily fish (sardines, mackerel, salmon) regularly, you should consider a good quality supplement with good levels of EPA and DHA (from fish or algae).

Dairy

Should we be eating dairy or not? If you're looking to find the answer to this on Google, don't bother! You'll get tons of conflicting information, even among nutrition experts.

Dairy products have long been associated with higher levels of inflammation, heart disease and even increased cancer risk. But the evidence is not conclusive and often conflicting, and there is robust evidence that dairy consumption actually lowers the risk of heart disease, type 2 diabetes, obesity and colorectal cancer. Interestingly, there's no evidence it increases your cholesterol levels.

Confusing, right? The truth is that the relationship between dairy consumption and health is complex and varied, depending on the type of dairy products, and individual factors such as genetics, ethnicity, overall diet and health status.

Overall, if you're not intolerant to dairy, and you choose the right types, dairy is going to be a healthy choice.

Here's what to focus on:

- **Fermented dairy:** e.g. quality cheese (various types), live natural yoghurt, kefir – nutrient-dense and great for your gut.
- **Grass-fed butter (no spreads or tubs!):** rich in fat-soluble vitamins.
- **Full fat over low fat:** fat contains all the key nutrients, keeps blood sugar stable and helps keep you full. Only choose low fat if you don't metabolise fat well (learn more about DNA testing in Part 3).

If you are dairy-free, watch out for hidden additives in dairy-free 'milks' and yoghurts, such as oils (rapeseed or veg oils), thickeners such as carrageenan and gums, lecithin and natural flavourings – the less ingredients the better. And be aware of the carb and protein profile of different products (e.g. oat milk has a much higher glycaemic index than almond or coconut milks).

Lastly, it's important to recognise that we all metabolise and absorb fats (and other nutrients) differently. Factors such as your genetic profile, lifestyle and health history play a significant role. Additionally, issues with fat digestion and absorption can arise from nutrient deficiencies, underlying gut infections, inflammation, food sensitivities, stress and lifestyle choices. So, it's important to be mindful of the total amount of fat in your diet.

The wonders of olive oil
Good-quality olive oil is a must-have in your healthy ageing pantry! A staple of the Mediterranean diet for centuries, olive oil has long been revered for its taste and health benefits. Hippocrates, the 'father of medicine', is known to have called it "the great healer".

Rich in monounsaturated fats, particularly oleic acid, olive oil has many science-backed health benefits including:

- **Heart health:** Just two tablespoons of extra virgin olive oil (EVOO) have been shown to help lower cholesterol (reducing LDL oxidation and increasing HDL), lower blood pressure and reduce the risk of blood clots.
- **Blood sugar control:** Monounsaturated fats are known to help with insulin sensitivity and blood sugar control. In one study, people at risk of diabetes took two tablespoons of EVOO a day for 18 months and reduced their fasting blood levels to normal.
- **Anti-inflammatory:** Several compounds present in EVOO, such as monounsaturated fats (MUFAs) and polyphenols, are known for their anti-inflammatory

properties. EVOO may help relieve pain associated with inflammation, such as arthritis.

- **Antioxidant:** EVOO is rich in antioxidants, including vitamin E (tocopherol), compounds known for their ability to combat oxidative stress.
- **Brain health:** The polyphenol compounds in EVOO have been linked to improved brain function and a lower risk of neurodegenerative diseases like Alzheimer's. A recent 30-year study involving over 90,000 individuals showed that even a small amount of olive oil every day may reduce the risk of dementia-related death by approximately 28%, regardless of the overall healthiness of your diet!
- **Bone health:** EVOO helps to preserve bone density, vital for reducing the risk of osteoporosis.

Quality matters: choosing the right olive oil

Just like fresh fruit juice, the health benefits of olive oil are most potent when it's fresh and minimally processed. Here's why quality matters:

- **Freshness:** Olive oil is richest in antioxidants and beneficial compounds right after it's harvested. Over time, these properties can diminish. Choosing oils from the latest harvest ensures you're getting the most out of its health benefits.
- **Processing:** The way olive oil is processed can significantly impact its quality. EVOO obtained through cold pressing without chemicals or high heat, retains the maximum amount of nutrients and antioxidants. Small batches from single origin farms ensure the best quality and freshness.
- **Storage:** Proper storage is key. Olive oil should be kept in a cool, dark place to preserve its quality. Make sure the bottle is dark too. Exposure to light and heat can lead to oxidation, diminishing its health benefits.

Avoid mass-produced, processed or old olive oil. Here are some things to remember:

- Choose EVOO over plain olive oil
- Choose EVOO in dark bottles and store in a dark cupboard or pantry
- Check the origin – avoid blends, go for single origin brands (e.g. from one Italian farm)
- Check the harvest date – the most recent the better

Integrating EVOO into your daily diet is easy and delicious. It's safe to cook with as it's very stable at most temperatures. You can also drizzle it over your meals, use it in baking or simply dip your bread in it.

For my favourite brands, head to the website for links and exclusive discounts: www.happyhormonesforlife.com/recommendations

CARBOHYDRATES
Carbohydrates often get a bad rap, mainly due to the impact that refined carbohydrates can have on your weight, blood sugar, insulin and inflammation.

But carbs are not your enemy! Unless you have a specific health condition, or you do better on a keto-style diet, most of us need to eat healthy carbs like fruit, vegetables, beans, pulses and whole grains.

Carbohydrates come in many forms, and their impact on our health and longevity can vary a lot. High-glycaemic index carbs, like refined sugars and processed grains, are linked to a higher risk of chronic diseases like diabetes, heart disease and cancer. On the other hand, low-glycaemic index carbs, such as whole grains, legumes, and vegetables, are good for overall health. They are a primary source of energy, breaking down into glucose, which fuels everything from your muscles to your brain.

Good-quality carbs also offer essential nutrients. Whole grains, for example, are rich in B vitamins that support metabolic health, and fruits and vegetables deliver vital vitamins, minerals, and antioxidants. Prebiotics and dietary fibre are other crucial components of healthy carbs. Prebiotic fibres, such as inulin, fructo-oligosaccharides (FOS) and galacto-oligosaccharides (GOS), feed the beneficial gut bacteria in our microbiomes. Food sources rich in prebiotic carbohydrates include onion, chicory, garlic, asparagus, banana (containing FOS), and legumes and beans (containing GOS). Found in foods like whole grains, fruits and vegetables, fibre aids in digestion and can help regulate blood sugar levels, reducing the risk of type 2 diabetes.

I hear all too often from women on very low-carb diets that they feel more depressed and irritable. That's because carbs have a role in your brain health, especially the production of serotonin. And while ketogenic diets can support weight loss and other health benefits, they can also lead to fatigue, nutritional deficiencies, more hot flushes and muscle loss in some women.

Your own relationship with carbs will depend on your genetics, lifestyle and health status. However, in general, opt for low-glycaemic complex carbohydrates over refined versions, and eat protein and healthy fats along with your carbs to slow down the release of glucose into the bloodstream.

Healthy carb swaps

- Wheat pasta for brown rice, lentil or chickpea pasta
- Spaghetti for courgetti, rice noodles or buckwheat noodles
- White rice for brown/wild rice, quinoa, black rice or cauliflower 'rice'
- Mashed potato for cauliflower, celeriac or sweet potato mash
- Tortilla wraps for little gem lettuce wraps, or low-carb seeded wraps
- Crisps for nuts, seeds, kale chips, seed crackers

- Cereal for low-sugar granola, chia pots or overnight oats
- Biscuits for oatcakes
- White or brown bread for good quality sourdough or flaxbread

Micronutrients

Micronutrients are the vitamins and minerals that, although required in smaller amounts, play a massive role in our overall health, especially as we age. Think of them as the unsung heroes that support everything from our immune system to cellular repair.

Unlike macronutrients, which provide the energy we need to function, micronutrients facilitate a host of physiological processes that are integral to healthy ageing. They're pivotal in supporting brain health, maintaining strong bones and even regulating our hormones.

B vitamins

Your B vitamins are vital for energy, mood, detoxification, hormone transport, brain function and so much more:

Vitamin B1 (thiamine): Needed to convert carbohydrates to energy. You will definitely need this one if you're low in energy.
- **Best food sources:** vegetables, nuts, seeds, beans, lentils, oats.
- **Best supplement form:** thiamin mononitrate or thiamin hydrochloride.

Vitamin B2 (riboflavin): Helps to metabolise carbs and essential fatty acids into energy sources and has a vital role to play in liver detoxification and immune health. It can also be helpful for headaches/migraines, acne and muscle cramps.
- **Best food sources:** green leafy veg, chicken, fish, soy, natural yoghurt, eggs.
- **Best supplement form:** riboflavin or riboflavin-5-phosphate.

Vitamin B3 (niacin): Another one for energy production but also vital for your thyroid, blood sugar, mood, nerve function and cell membranes. It can also help to lower cholesterol (check with your doctor before taking it for that).
- **Best food sources:** meat, fish, brown rice, peanuts, seeds, almonds, seaweed.
- **Best supplement form:** nicotinamide (non flushing).

Vitamin B5 (pantothenic acid): Vital for the production of adrenal hormones, especially important for those under a lot of stress. It's also needed for the production of your sex hormones.
- **Best food sources**: avocados, mushrooms, soy, bananas, cabbage, broccoli, kale, brown rice, eggs, poultry, sweet potatoes, natural yoghurt.
- **Best supplement form:** calcium pantothenate.

Vitamin B6 (pyridoxine): Your building block for protein and DNA. Great for mood as it stimulates serotonin, and essential in detoxification of steroid hormones such as oestrogen (helps to reduce risk of oestrogen driven cancers). Key roles in brain health and immune function too!
- **Best food sources**: spinach, walnuts, eggs, fish, poultry, beans, potatoes, bananas, chickpeas.
- **Best supplement form:** pyridoxine HCL or pyridoxal-5-phosphate.

Vitamin B7 (biotin): as well as metabolising your carbs, protein and fats into energy, biotin has also been shown to help with blood sugar balance and your skin, hair and nails.
- **Best food sources:** vegetables, nuts, seeds, beans, lentils, oats.
- **Best supplement form:** biotin.

Vitamin B9 (folic acid or folate): Critical for detoxification pathways, breaking down homocysteine which can cause inflammation. It's also really vital for mood and protecting the foetus in pregnancy.
- **Best food sources:** asparagus, dark leafy greens, bananas, beans, peas, peanuts, citrus fruits.

- **Best supplement form:** 5-methyltetrahydrofolate or calcium-L-methylfolate.

Vitamin B12 (cobalamin): Critical for energy production, nerve function and brain health. Up to 15% of adults aged 65 and older in the UK are deficient in vitamin B12! Symptoms can include fatigue, dizzy spells, muscle weakness, low mood, confusion, loss of appetite. Get tested if you have any of these symptoms.
- **Best food sources:** animal products (dairy, fish, meat, eggs). Vegans or vegetarians should get tested to identify any deficiencies.
- **Best supplement form:** methylcobalamin.

Vitamin A
Vitamin A is essential for healthy vision, immune function, skin health, reproductive health, and ensures proper functioning of the heart, lungs and kidneys. Retinol form of vitamin A is directly usable by the body, whereas the provitamin compound of beta-carotene needs to be converted into retinol.
- **Best food sources:** liver, oily fish, dairy products, and egg yolks for retinol, and brightly coloured fruits and vegetables like carrots, sweet potatoes, spinach and kale for beta-carotene.
- **Best supplement form:** retinol palmitate or retinyl acetate, beta-carotene or a combination.

Vitamin C
A powerful antioxidant, vitamin C supports immune function, skin, collagen production for healthy skin and tissues, and neutralises harmful free radicals in the body.
- **Best food sources**: kiwis, bell peppers, citrus fruits, berries, pineapple, mango, kale, spinach.
- **Best supplement form**: vitamin C ascorbic acid, or liposomal vitamin C.

Vitamin E

Another powerful antioxidant, vitamin E protects cells from oxidative damage, supports the immune system, skin and eye health, and may reduce the risk of chronic diseases like heart disease.

- **Best food sources:** nuts and seeds (especially almonds and sunflower seeds), green leafy vegetables (especially spinach and kale), avocados, oily fish, red bell peppers.
- **Best supplement form:** d-alpha-tocopherol or mixed tocopherols.

Vitamin K

Essential for blood clotting, supporting bone health and regulating inflammation. Vitamin K2 is particularly beneficial for bone and cardiovascular health.

- **Best food sources:** green leafy vegetables (such as kale, spinach, and broccoli), Brussels sprouts, green beans, and fermented foods like natto.
- **Best supplement form:** vitamin K1 (phylloquinone) and vitamin K2 (menaquinone).

Minerals

- **Calcium:** Essential for strong bones and teeth, muscle function, and nerve signalling.
- **Magnesium:** Important for muscle and nerve function, energy production, bone health, sleep and maintaining a healthy immune system.
- **Potassium:** Regulates fluid balance, muscle contractions, and nerve signals, and supports heart health.
- **Sodium:** Essential for maintaining fluid balance, nerve function and muscle contractions.
- **Iron:** Necessary for the production of haemoglobin, which carries oxygen in the blood, and supports energy metabolism.
- **Zinc:** Vital for immune function, wound healing, DNA synthesis, stomach acid and cell division.
- **Selenium:** Key antioxidant, supports thyroid function, and boosts the immune system

- **Copper:** Involved in red blood cell production, maintaining healthy nerves and immune function, and forming collagen.
- **Iodine:** Essential for thyroid health and brain function.
- **Manganese:** Important for bone formation, metabolism and antioxidant defence.
- **Boron:** Supports bone health, brain function and the metabolism of minerals such as calcium and magnesium.

By incorporating a varied and colourful diet rich in fruits, vegetables, protein, nuts, seeds, legumes, healthy fats and complex carbohydrates, you'll cover most of these micronutrient bases. But I would recommend supplementation of a good-quality multivitamin and mineral to ensure you are getting the required amounts.

Vitamin D

One vitamin you won't get enough of in your diet is vitamin D. And it's a crucial part of your healthy ageing toolkit! You can get small amounts of it from animal foods, such as egg yolks, meat, oily fish and dairy, but it's not enough to keep your levels in the optimal range.

Did you know that vitamin D is actually a hormone, not a vitamin? It has receptors in nearly every cell in your body, and growing evidence shows that its role extends far beyond merely supporting your bones.

Vital for immunity, brain function and mood, vitamin D has also been shown to slow down cellular ageing, reduce inflammation, enhance DNA repair and influence genomic stability.

Vitamin D benefits include:

- **Immune system:** Vitamin D supports your immune system and helps fight infections, which might explain why colds and flu are more common in winter when there's less sunlight.
- **Autoimmune protection:** Deficiency in vitamin D has been linked to various autoimmune conditions, such as multiple sclerosis (MS), Crohn's disease, rheumatoid arthritis and Hashimoto's thyroiditis.
- **Cancer protection:** Increasing evidence suggests a connection between vitamin D deficiency and certain cancers, including breast, prostate and colon cancer. Some studies suggest that adequate vitamin D levels could cut the rates of these cancers by up to 50%.
- **Bone and muscle health:** Vitamin D regulates calcium levels and the activity of bone-building cells, helping to prevent conditions like rickets and osteoporosis.
- **Brain health**: It plays a crucial role in neurological health, influencing mood and cognitive function. It is known to lower neurodegenerative disease risk through its anti-inflammatory and antioxidant properties.
- **Heart health:** Vitamin D helps prevent calcium build-up in the arteries, normalises blood pressure and reduces inflammation.
- **Skin health:** It can prevent excessive cell proliferation, which is beneficial for conditions like psoriasis and eczema.
- **Blood sugar balance and insulin control:** Vitamin D aids in regulating blood sugar levels and preventing insulin resistance.
- **Longevity:** Low vitamin D levels are associated with increased mortality rates, indicating its role in promoting a longer life. One study showed that taking 4000IU per day reduced biological age by 1.85 years in just 16 weeks!

How to get enough Vitamin D:

- **Get sun exposure,** without sunscreen, for as long as you can without burning.
- **Get tested** for optimal levels (not just 'adequate').
- **Supplement with vitamin D3** during the winter months or all year round if you are not exposing your skin to the sun.
- **Supplement with D3 co-factor vitamins and minerals:** K2, magnesium, vitamin A, boron, zinc.

Jump to Activate for more info on supplements.

Plant nutrients

Now let's talk about the power of plants. One of the commonalities of the Blue Zones, the regions in the world with the most centenarians, is their high consumption of plant foods.

Phytonutrients are compounds found in plants that have significant health benefits. These powerful substances are not just pigments that make fruits and vegetables taste good and look colourful; they're also potent antioxidants that fight off free radicals, reducing oxidative stress and lowering the risk of chronic disease.

Plenty of studies have shown that a Mediterranean-based diet, rich in fruits, vegetables, legumes, nuts, seeds, whole grains, olive oil, herbs and spices, all key sources of phytonutrients, is correlated with better health outcomes in older adults.

Additionally, plants are by far the biggest source of fibre. Fibre keeps our digestive system running smoothly by adding bulk to the stool and preventing constipation, while also working wonders for our heart by lowering cholesterol levels and reducing the risk of heart disease and stroke. Plus, fibre helps with blood sugar control, weight management and it's crucial for a healthy gut microbiome, all of which help lower our risk of chronic disease as we get older.

Getting a diverse range of plant foods in your diet is going to give you plenty of plant nutrients, and also keep your microbiome happy (your bugs love variety!). While 'five a day' of fruit and veg has generally been the UK dietary advice for years, we should really be targeting ten portions a day if we want to live longer. A study published in 2017 concluded that this could potentially prevent nearly 7.8 million premature deaths!

Geek Alert

Here is a selection of common phytonutrients and their benefits:

Polyphenols: These encompass a wide range of phytonutrients found in berries, cherries, grapes and other fruits and vegetables, as well as in tea and coffee. They are particularly plentiful in herbs and spices such as cloves, rosemary, thyme, oregano, cinnamon, sage, peppermint, basil, parsley, turmeric, ginger, cumin and black pepper. Polyphenols have antioxidant and anti-inflammatory properties. They've been linked to a lower risk of chronic diseases such as cardiovascular disease and certain cancers.

Flavonoids: Found in fruits, vegetables and beverages like tea, these compounds have antioxidant, anti-inflammatory, and anti-cancer properties. They're known to improve heart health and may help reduce the risk of neurodegenerative diseases.

Carotenoids: Present in colourful fruits and vegetables like carrots, sweet potatoes and spinach, these compounds can convert to vitamin A in the body. They are known for their antioxidant activity and have been shown to improve eye health and boost the immune system. Lycopene from tomatoes can help protect against stroke and heart disease.

Glucosinolates: Found in cruciferous vegetables like broccoli, Brussels sprouts and cabbage, these compounds have potential to detoxify carcinogens and inhibit tumour growth.

Lignans: Present in seeds, particularly flaxseeds, as well as grains and vegetables, lignans have antioxidant properties and may contribute to heart health. They also have potential benefits for bone health.

Saponins: Found in beans and legumes, these compounds have antioxidant and immune-boosting properties and may help lower cholesterol.

Phytosterols: Present in nuts and seeds, they are structurally similar to cholesterol and can help in lowering LDL cholesterol levels.

Allicin: Found in garlic, onions and leeks, allicin has anti-inflammatory, antioxidant and antimicrobial properties. It has been shown to improve heart health and strengthen the immune system.

Phenolic acids: Found in a variety of plant-based foods, including fruits, vegetables, whole grains, nuts and seeds. Known for strong antioxidant and anti-inflammatory properties.

Limonoids: Present in citrus fruits like lemons, oranges and grapefruits, limonoids are known for their antioxidant and anti-cancer properties.

Anthocyanins: These are found in red, purple or blue fruits like berries and grapes. They are powerful antioxidants and have been linked to improved heart health and brain function.

Lutein and zeaxanthin: Found in dark green leafy vegetables, these phytonutrients are crucial for eye health and have been shown to reduce the risk of macular degeneration, a common issue in ageing populations.

Ellagic acid: Found in nuts and berries, especially raspberries and strawberries, ellagic acid has been studied for its anti-cancer and antioxidant properties.

Quercetin: Found in apples, onions, grapes, parsley, sage and tea, this antioxidant can help fight inflammation and lower blood pressure.

Sulforaphane: Found primarily in cruciferous vegetables like broccoli, Brussels sprouts, and cabbage, sulforaphane has potent anti-cancer and anti-inflammatory properties. Studies have shown it to be effective in detoxifying harmful substances and protecting cells from damage, both important factors in healthy ageing.

Isoflavones: Commonly found in soy products, isoflavones are known for their antioxidant, anti-inflammatory, and anti-cancer properties. They can also act as phytoestrogens, which can help to reduce some menopausal symptoms.

Capsaicin: Found in chilli peppers, capsaicin has been researched for its benefits in reducing pain and inflammation, boosting metabolism, and even improving longevity.

Betalains: Found in beets and Swiss chard, these phytonutrients have strong antioxidant and anti-inflammatory effects.

Tannins: Found in tea and some fruits like grapes and pomegranates, tannins have antioxidant properties and can improve gut health.

Resveratrol: Found in grapes, red wine and berries, resveratrol is known for its antioxidant and anti-inflammatory properties. It's often touted for its potential to improve cardiovascular health and increase longevity. Some studies have even indicated that it can activate sirtuins, proteins that help to regulate cellular health and ageing.

Fisetin: A particular flavonoid found in various fruits and vegetables, including strawberries, apples, grapes and cucumbers, fisetin has anti-inflammatory, antioxidant, and neuroprotective properties. It's also been shown to clear those 'zombie' senescent cells, which can contribute to inflammation and other age-related diseases.

Epigallocatechins (EGCG): One of the most abundant and biologically active compounds in green tea and is known for its numerous potential health benefits.

Curcumin: A naturally occurring polyphenolic compound found in the root of the turmeric plant, known for its vibrant yellow colour and anti-inflammatory, anti-cancer, and antioxidant properties.

Remember, the real power of these phytonutrients comes from their synergy – eating a colourful variety of fruits, vegetables, herbs, spices and herbal teas, will provide the most comprehensive health benefits.

Anti-nutrients in plant foods

Not everyone will respond well to lots of fibre, legumes, grains and nuts. Many of these foods contain anti-nutrients, compounds that plants use as defence mechanisms, which can sometimes interfere with nutrient absorption in humans. These include phytates, lectins, oxalates, tannins and saponins, which are normally broken down by our gut, but in some people can cause uncomfortable symptoms such as bloating, indigestion and other digestive issues. They can also inhibit the absorption of nutrients like calcium, zinc, magnesium and iron, as well as vital enzymes and proteins.

Some foods to watch out for include legumes (especially kidney beans, soy, lentils, chickpeas), spinach (swap for kale or other greens in smoothies), gluten-containing grains, nuts (e.g. almonds, walnuts) and some fruits. Soaking, fermenting and cooking can help reduce these compounds, but if you suffer any digestive symptoms, do avoid or seek support for your gut health.

Phytoestrogens

Nature has provided plant compounds that can help support our oestrogen levels, both in the manufacture of HRT (body identical brands are mostly made from yams), but also in our diet.

Phytoestrogens are natural plant compounds that are structurally similar to human oestrogen and can mimic the action of oestrogen in the body. Although they are only about one-thousandth as potent as human oestrogen (and body identical HRT), research shows they can help reduce menopausal symptoms and also protect against heart disease and osteoporosis.

In fact, we know that women in Asian countries, such as Japan, who consume traditional diets rich in soy and other phytoestrogen-containing foods, tend to experience fewer menopausal symptoms compared to women in Western countries. Research so far is only observational but many believe that the phytoestrogens in their diet are one of the reasons for the disparity.

There are many types of phytoestrogens in plants, but the most significant for menopause symptoms are the isoflavones, most commonly found in soy products, and lignans, most commonly found in flaxseeds.

Soy: It's important to avoid any genetically modified (GM) soy, so always buy organic, and avoid added sugar or oils where possible. Here are some ideas:

- organic unsweetened soy milk
- organic soy natural yoghurt
- organic tofu and tempeh
- edamame beans
- miso

Some people are intolerant to soy, so if you have any reaction when eating soy, do stop! You can always try supplements.

Flaxseeds (or linseeds) = 1–2 tbsp per day (milled to get the lignans)

- sprinkle on yoghurt
- put in your smoothie
- make some flaxseed crackers
- sprinkle on salads or soups

Other sources of phytoestrogens:

- chickpeas and hummus
- sesame seeds
- pumpkin seeds
- legumes
- dried apricots
- alfalfa sprouts
- mung beans
- rye bran

AND … dark chocolate (yay!).

If you can't get enough phytoestrogens in your diet, certain supplements can help, in particular ones containing isoflavones (red clover extract is a particularly good one).

Longevity superfoods

There are a few specific foods that deserve a special mention when it comes to healthy ageing.

Berries: Berries are celebrated for their high levels of antioxidants, flavonoids, and polyphenols, all of which help combat oxidative stress and inflammation—two key drivers of ageing. Studies show that those who regularly eat berries have a 21% lower risk of mortality from any cause. Cranberry lovers benefit the most, with a 31% lower risk, while regular blueberry eaters enjoy a 21% reduction, and strawberry fans see a 14% decrease. For best results, choose organic berries to avoid exposure to pesticides.

Beans: A staple of each of the Blue Zone diets, beans are a powerhouse of nutrients, including fibre, protein, folate and key minerals like iron, potassium and magnesium. Research shows that for every 20g of beans consumed daily, there's a 7% drop in mortality risk. Opt for organic beans where possible, and note that canned varieties tend to have lower levels of lectins, making them easier to digest for some people.

Nuts and seeds: Packed with healthy fats, fibre, protein, vitamins and minerals, nuts and seeds offer numerous health benefits, including reducing your risk of heart disease, diabetes, dementia and certain cancers. They have even been shown to increase the length of your telomeres and reduce cell senescence! Incorporate a mix of almonds, Brazil nuts, walnuts, chia seeds, flaxseeds, and more. Keep them as unprocessed as possible and remember that peanuts, while technically a legume, share many of these benefits.

Cruciferous vegetables: This group of veggies belong to the Brassica family and include broccoli, Brussels sprouts, cabbage, cauliflower, kale, bok choy, radish (and horseradish), rocket, watercress, turnips, collard greens and Swiss chard. They are rich in fibre (100 calories' worth provides about 25–40% of your daily fibre requirement), key vitamins, minerals and phytonutrients, including antioxidants, glucosinolates, sulforaphane and indole-3-carbinol. Research has linked these compounds to improved heart health, brain function, hormone balance, detoxification, cancer prevention and longevity.

Eggs: The humble egg has a lot going for it when it comes to healthy ageing! Eggs offer high-quality protein and a range of essential nutrients like B vitamins, vitamin D, selenium, and phosphorus. One study found that replacing red meat with 50g of eggs per day can reduce total mortality by 8%. Don't skip the yolks—they're rich in choline, folate, and B12, which support DNA methylation and healthy ageing.

Olive oil: Often known as 'liquid gold', I like to think of olive oil as the elixir of healthy ageing. Skip back to the section on Fats if you missed all the details.

SMASH fish: An easy way to remember these types of fish, 'salmon, mackerel, anchovies, sardines, and herring', which are naturally high in omega-3 fats, and lowest in mercury levels. Great for heart and brain health, two of the systems we need to really protect as we age.

Gut-loving foods: As we've seen in Part 2, and later in Eliminate, our gut health is paramount to ageing well. Foods to support our gut include prebiotics (e.g. chicory root, garlic, onions, leeks, asparagus, bananas, artichokes, apples, flaxseeds), and probiotics (e.g. yoghurt, kefir, sauerkraut, kimchi, kombucha, sourdough bread, apple cider vinegar).

Chocolate, red wine and coffee: I'm a big believer that indulgences can be part of a healthy lifestyle when chosen wisely, so these 3 make my list!

- Dark chocolate - chocolate with high cocoa content (over 70%), contains several beneficial phytonutrients, including flavanols, polyphenols, theobromine and anandamide (known as the 'bliss' molecule!). These compounds help fend off oxidative stress and inflammation, improving heart health, mood regulation and cognitive function. More recently it's even been shown to help with healthy ageing, through supporting mitochondrial function and reducing zombie cells. It's also rich in magnesium, which is your body's relaxation mineral (no wonder we eat more chocolate when we're stressed!).

- Red wine - I've talked about the health risks of alcohol already, so why am I including red wine here? Because if you're like me and love a nice glass of good red, a little of what makes you happy sometimes does you more good than harm if you're sensible. While red wine contains beneficial phytonutrients including resveratrol, anthocyanins, quercetin, catechins, tannins and ellagic acid, it's a stretch to include it in any healthy eating protocol. However, if you do enjoy a glass, opt for high-quality, preferably organic, varieties and drink it with food (and friends!) to minimise any adverse effects.

- Coffee - another of my favourites, is rich in phytonutrients like chlorogenic acids and cafestol. Studies show that coffee can reduce the risk of diabetes, heart disease, and even extend telomere length! Opt for organic, low-mycotoxin brands and avoid sugary add-ins (a grande-size latte from Starbucks contains almost 18g of sugar, while the oat milk version has 28g of sugar!). Drinking coffee after breakfast, rather than on an empty stomach, helps prevent cortisol spikes.

Water

It's too obvious, right? We all know we should drink enough water. But are we actually DOING it?

Hydration goes beyond just drinking water; it involves providing your body with essential minerals like sodium, potassium, chloride, calcium and magnesium. These minerals are vital for brain function, mood, heart health, kidney health, digestion, skin, joints and internal vessel lubrication (yes, including your vagina!).

Additionally, they help cell repair, assist blood cells in nutrient transport, and even help keep cravings and hunger in check.

Symptoms of dehydration are hard to spot as they can resemble common menopause issues, so if you have any of these, make sure to properly hydrate yourself and see what happens. Some common signs to look out for include fatigue, headaches, dry mouth, dry eyes, dry skin, constipation, infrequent urination, dark-coloured urine, heart palpitations, brain fog and memory loss, mood swings, anxiety, depression, muscle cramps, confusion, dizziness and shortness of breath.

How much water we need will differ per person. We lose water in breathing, sweating and producing urine and you will need more if it's hot, you're sweating, exercising or if you're having hot flushes.

It's best and more accurate to find out how hydrated you are through the colour of your urine. You'll notice first thing in the morning, your urine is normally orange and then as you go through the day it should get lighter and lighter. You should be aiming for a yellow pale straw-like colour for full hydration.

Don't wait til you get thirsty! We lose our thirst perception from the age of 20 onwards, and by 70 we can lose it altogether and not realise we need to drink.

With all our medical advances, sometimes it's the basic things that we need to remember.

Here are some handy tips to make sure you're drinking enough water:

- Drink a large glass of water first thing in the morning to rehydrate you after your sleep.
- Fill a large bottle of water up in the morning and make sure you drink it all by bedtime.

- Drink before, during and after a workout.
- Get an app or set up some notifications to remind you to drink every hour.
- Try adding electrolytes (or sea salt) to your water for a quick hydration fix.
- Add flavour if it helps you drink more – e.g. slices of cucumber, mint leaves, berries (be careful of lemon/lime as this can damage your teeth enamel).
- Limit alcohol (try matching each drink with a glass of water and then more before bed).
- Coffee and tea do count – while the caffeine can have a diuretic effect (make you pee more), the water content will help you hydrate.
- Eat plenty of fruit and veg, especially celery, watermelon, cucumber, tomatoes – these add to your water intake.
- Include soups and smoothies in your diet.
- When you feel hungry and want a snack, often it's actually that the body is THIRSTY, and a large glass of water will do the job (and help you manage your weight too!). One study found that increased water consumption was linked to greater weight loss and fat loss in overweight and obese adults.

WHEN AND HOW TO EAT

We don't just need to watch WHAT we eat to age well. We also have to be mindful about WHEN and HOW we eat. Again, this will vary for every individual, your own unique metabolism, as well as your daily routine and lifestyle. The main thing is to do your own experimenting and see what works for you.

Timing of meals is a hotly debated topic amongst wellness experts. The old mantras of 'never skip breakfast', and 'eat little and often' have been swapped for 'time restricted eating' and 'no snacking'.

In truth, the research is pretty mixed on the best time to eat, with some people doing better eating earlier in the day, and others later. However, there is solid evidence that fasting in various formats is beneficial for most of us, whether that's just leaving bigger gaps between meals, or fasting for longer periods. I'll cover this in more detail in the Activate section of the EMBRACE protocol.

The HOW is important too. If we bolt our food down while responding to emails or scrolling social media, we are not going to digest it very well and we're more likely to overeat.

It's important to slow down, eat mindfully, appreciate your food and chew chew chew! This way your food gets properly digested as it moves through (avoiding bloating and indigestion), and your stomach has time to send the fullness signal to your brain so that you stop eating BEFORE you get too full. Studies suggest that it takes 20 minutes for those signals to work.

Okinawans (one of the Blue Zone regions) follow a time-honoured tradition dating back 2,500 years known as *'Hara hachi bu'*, which serves as a gentle reminder to practise mindful eating and to stop consuming food when their stomachs are approximately 80% full.

The Blue Zone centenarians also tend to eat together socially. Research shows that eating with others has been associated with improved eating habits, enhanced mental wellbeing and a lower risk of obesity.

Movement after eating can help improve insulin sensitivity, enhance glucose uptake by muscles and reduce postprandial glycemia, contributing to better blood sugar control. A short walk after eating is all you need (even if it's just round the house).

SUMMARY

- There's no one-size-fits-all diet. Stick to healthy principles and be your own experiment.
- Eat real foods, enough good-quality protein, healthy fats and complex carbohydrates
- Aim to fill half your plate with colourful diverse vegetables.
- Use good olive oil and drink plenty of water.
- Limit sugar, ultra-processed foods and alcohol.
- Nourish your gut; eat slowly, chew each mouthful, feed your microbiome and watch out for intolerances.
- Stop eating before you're 100% full, eat with others if you can and move after your meals.
- Experiment with timings and incorporate some form of fasting.
- Listen to your body and trust what it's telling you.

CHAPTER 7

M – MOVE daily

Modern life is unfortunately making us less active. A typical working day may look like this: you drive (or get the train) to work, spend hours at your desk, then drive back home and sink into the sofa for the evening. It's a routine many of us are familiar with. In fact, the average British person sits for 8.9 hours a day (according to Public Health England).

But it's a far cry from how our ancestors lived. In caveman days, sitting for prolonged periods was virtually unheard of. Physiologically, our bodies are not well-suited to inactivity. Research shows that excessive sitting is linked to a host of chronic diseases, including cardiovascular disease and type 2 diabetes.

And if you're sedentary for over 12 hours a day, you face a 38% increased risk of death compared to those with a daily sedentary time of eight hours, according to a study in the *British Journal of Sports Medicine.*

What's worse is that prolonged sitting can even wipe out the benefits of any exercise you do. That means, if you're exercising for an hour, but sitting for the rest of the day, it might not even count!

The good news is that these risks are much reduced through daily movement, which is why moving and physical activity is a vital part of the EMBRACE protocol.

Exercise has a host of benefits: it revs up your antioxidant systems, sharpens your brain function and lifts your mood. It helps with gut diversity, hormone balance, stress, heart, immune and liver function. It can even add a little spice to your love life!

And when it comes to longevity, exercise has been shown to lengthen your telomeres, amp up your metabolic pathways, and engage those anti-ageing sirtuins. It can support your mitochondria, reduce inflammation, trigger autophagy and even reset some of the age-related changes in your DNA.

There's a fine line, however. Exercise is a natural stressor for your body, and as always, there's good stress and bad stress. The right amount of stress from exercise prompts your body to adapt and become more resilient. However, too much stress from exercise can deplete your adrenals and make you feel worse. If pushing yourself to the limit at the gym, in a spin class, or on long runs leaves you feeling drained and depleted afterwards, it's usually a sign that you need to adopt a gentler approach.

Working out the type and amount of exercise that's right for you depends on various factors, such as your fitness level, health, lifestyle and personal preferences.

The trick is to find a routine that suits your abilities, brings enjoyment, and makes you feel good. For those with limited mobility, even gentle stretching or small adapted movements can be very effective. Where possible, I'd recommend you look at a mixture of activity that incorporates the three Ss – Sweat, Strengthen and Stretch, plus pelvic floor exercises and general daily movement to suit.

SWEAT

Sweating is more than just a sign you're working hard during exercise. Not only does it help to regulate your temperature, sweating is also a key function of your immune system.

The presence of antimicrobial peptides in sweat helps to maintain the skin's microbiome balance and protect against skin infections. Additionally, sweating during physical activity can help to flush out toxins and pathogens from the skin.

And the endorphins of a good sweat are hard to beat, so it's great for your mood.

Ways to break a sweat:

- **Brisk walking (or walking uphill):** Free and accessible, walking is the easiest way for most of us to get our heart rate up and a sweat on. See the upcoming section on walking for all the amazing health benefits.
- **Running or jogging:** While the cardiovascular aspect of running or jogging are advantageous, it can be tough on the joints, especially the knees and hips. If you're in any discomfort or pain, it's crucial to listen to your body and consider lower-impact alternatives like walking or swimming.
- **Swimming:** If you still crave the cardio high, but have problems with your joints, swimming could be for you. One study involving 62 perimenopausal women found that swimming three times per week improved glucose control and insulin sensitivity. The study also found that shorter high intensity intermittent swimming was more beneficial than swimming at low intensity for one hour. So, if you fancy trying HIIT but don't think your joints could take it, try HIIT swimming instead.
  If it's accessible to you, a wild swim in nature gives you the added benefit of cold exposure, which we know is great for your health.
- **Cycling:** Cycling is another fantastic way for us to reap cardiovascular benefits while being easier on the joints. It's a great way to improve lung capacity and circulation, while building muscle tone, particularly in the lower body. Whether you're cycling outdoors or opting for a stationary bike indoors, it can be easily modified to suit your fitness level.
- **Tennis and badminton:** According to one study, these two sports are particularly beneficial for longevity, with

badminton potentially adding an average of 6.2 years to one's life compared to an inactive person, while tennis can add nearly a decade! The principles of hand-eye coordination and playing in a social setting might also apply to table tennis, squash and pickleball.

- **Stair climbing:** This simple activity engages multiple muscle groups, helps strengthen your legs, and improves cardiovascular and bone health. It's also a practical way to sneak in exercise without requiring extra time or specialised equipment.
- **Elliptical machine:** If you have access to an elliptical machine, it mimics the motions of jogging or walking but with much less stress on your knees, hips and back. Plus, you're also engaging your upper body muscles like shoulders, back and arms.
- **Rowing:** Rowing (in a boat or on a machine) provides a superb total-body workout that targets both upper and lower body while being easy on the joints.
- **Dancing or dance-based aerobics:** If you're not fond of traditional aerobic exercise, dancing can be a great alternative. Stick on your favourite track, and dance like nobody's watching! Or go to a Zumba or dance class if you need some motivation.
- **Aqua aerobics:** A fun, low-impact workout that improves cardiovascular fitness, muscle strength and flexibility while reducing stress on the joints. A great activity for injury recovery too.
- **High intensity interval training (HIIT):** If you are in good health, your joints are sound and your stress levels aren't too high, then HIIT is a great way to improve fitness and burn fat. Another huge plus point is that it doesn't take up too much time.

STRENGTHEN

Strength training is one of the best defences against the effects of ageing – which is why I'm finally taking this one seriously on a personal level.

As we saw in Part 1, we are fighting hard to stand still in the race against muscle loss after 40.

Not only does strength work help offset this loss, it helps to stoke your metabolism and reduce fat stores, while also improving brain health and mood.

JJ Virgin, a nutritionist in the US, says muscle is like 'metabolic spanx' – it holds everything together! Muscle requires more energy to exist, so it burns more calories from your food. It's also like a 'sugar sponge', as it's an alternative to your fat cells for storing carbohydrates.

Strength training helps maintain bone density and reduces the risk of osteoporosis, while also promoting proper posture and joint stability. Additionally, it improves overall mobility, lowering the risk of injury and falls. It also stimulates anabolic hormones like testosterone and growth hormone, which can regulate fat stores and weight, while also improving glucose metabolism and reducing the risk of insulin resistance.

And there's good evidence for longevity. A key study in 2022 found that doing any amount of resistance training, like lifting weights or using resistance bands can lower your risk of dying from any cause, heart disease or cancer by 15%!

Remember those 'zombie' cells that don't go away and cause faster ageing? Strength training is a great way to fight them. Resistance exercise causes slight tears in the muscle tissue, which is why you might feel sore the day after lifting weights. As the muscle tissues break down, immune cells migrate to the site where repair is needed, wiping away any zombie cells while they're at it.

So, if we want to age the best we can, it's vital that we incorporate some form of strength and resistance training into our routines.

What's interesting is that you don't need to do a lot of it – just about an hour of resistance training each week can give you the maximum benefits in terms of reducing these risks. So, even a small amount of this kind of exercise can make a big difference to your health.

There are so many ways that you can add strength training into your routine from incorporating a set of weights or resistance bands into your exercise kit at home, to using that park bench as a tricep dip stop.

How to include strength training into your daily routine without needing to go to the gym:

- **Bodyweight exercises at home:** Use your own body weight as resistance. E.g. push-ups, squats, lunges, tricep dips, planks and burpees.
- **Resistance bands**: Invest in a set of resistance bands. They're portable and can provide varying levels of resistance for different muscle groups.
- **Use household items:** Get creative with everyday household items as makeshift weights. You can use water bottles, canned goods, or even a backpack filled with books to add resistance to exercises like bicep curls, lateral raises, and squats.
- **Stairs:** Run up and down your stairs a few times a day to work your legs.
- **Daily chores with intent:** While doing household chores like gardening, housework or carrying groceries, focus on engaging your muscles.
- **Exercise snacks:** Throughout the day, take short breaks to do quick strength-building exercises, e.g. do some squats while you're brushing your teeth, or pick up some dumb-bells while you're waiting for the kettle to boil.
- **Pilates and yoga:** Both these practices incorporate poses and movement designed to improve your strength. Attend a class or join an online programme.
- **Resistance training apps:** Consider using apps that guide you through bodyweight or resistance-band workouts. These apps often provide structured routines and timers to keep you on track.

Remember to start gradually and focus on proper form to prevent injuries. It's also a good idea to consult with a fitness professional or physical therapist to create a personalised strength-training plan that suits your specific goals and needs.

Inspirational women: Kim Rahir

Kim, who I had the pleasure of interviewing on my Happy Hormones Podcast, is a 60-year-old mother of three with a fascinating story to tell. She was diagnosed with MS at the age of 50 and decided to start strength training alongside her treatment to regain a feeling of power and control.

As she got stronger, she got better and today she has no sign of MS in her body. Not only that, in 2023, she became European Champion in Masters Weightlifting in her age and weight category. Her journey inspired her to leave her career in journalism in her 50s and become a health coach for middle-aged women – with a big focus on reactivating and rebuilding muscle.

Kim's secret: Focus on the best you can do right now and create momentum with small wins.

Listen to the full episode on the Happy Hormones podcast (ep. 144)

STRETCH

Once you start building muscles, it's really important to stretch them out. Mobility, balance, strength, fitness and flexibility are all equally key to healthy ageing.

Regular stretching offers numerous benefits, particularly as you age. Being able to move your joints freely and with control not only prevents injury and falls, but also lets you handle the everyday tasks of life, keeps you independent for longer and able to take part in activities that bring you joy and keep you socially connected.

Stretching also alleviates muscle stiffness, and helps you maintain good posture, reducing the risk of back pain and improving balance and coordination. It stimulates blood circulation, contributing to cardiovascular health, and provides stress relief, benefiting mental wellbeing.

My two favourite ways of staying mobile, flexible and strong are yoga and Pilates. They both have multiple benefits. I try to do a bit of both because I just feel so good afterwards – relaxed, centred and standing that little bit taller.

Tips for yoga and Pilates:

- Try different classes (online or in person, yoga and/or Pilates). Don't give up because you didn't enjoy the class. Find another class or teacher. Keep looking, when you find the right one, you'll know it.
- It doesn't matter if you're not flexible. A good teacher will give you options according to your ability. Don't compare yourself to others – do your best and you'll be fine.

Lots of people think exercise should be hard or intense to be any good for you. Research suggests otherwise, and especially for women in midlife.

If yoga or Pilates is not for you, try Tai Chi It offers numerous benefits for individuals with limited mobility. Its gentle movements and emphasis on balance and flexibility can improve range of motion, enhance stability and promote overall wellbeing.

Health benefits of yoga and Pilates

- **Stress:** Mindful breathing and focus used in both yoga and Pilates has been shown to reduce cortisol levels.
- **Anxiety and depression**: Regular practice has been shown in several studies to reduce feelings of anxiety and depression.

- **Heart health:** From increasing circulation to lowering blood pressure and cholesterol, both are great for your heart.
- **Pain:** Studies show that yoga and Pilates can relieve pain in people with carpal tunnel and osteoarthritis, so it's also likely to help with other pain too.
- **Bones:** As it is weight bearing, one study showed just 12 minutes of yoga a day improved bone density in spine and legs, helping to prevent osteoporosis.
- **Sleep:** Evidence shows that regular practice can increase sleep quality and duration, and even increase secretion of melatonin, your sleep hormone.
- **Flexibility, balance, strength and posture:** Both practices help you improve all of these.
- **Breathing and lung function:** Practising regular yogic and Pilates breathing can help improve lung capacity.
- **Migraines:** Studies have shown potential improvement in migraine symptoms after regular practice.
- **Immune system:** Research shows that regular practice can affect gene expression of your white blood cells to better fight infection.
- **Brain function:** Yoga has been shown to help with brain fog and processing information.

CORE AND PELVIC FLOOR

Looking after your core and pelvic floor is no longer about having a six pack of abs (although go for it if that's your thing!). These muscles provide stability, support and control for the entire body, helping to prevent issues such as back pain, incontinence, pelvic organ prolapse and maintaining mobility and quality of life as you age.

Oestrogen protects the whole pelvic floor region, so when levels decline, it can result in the GSM symptoms we discussed in Part 2; namely dry and thin vaginal walls, pain and irritation, bladder issues and risk of prolapse. It's especially important if you've had children or abdominal surgery, to include care for these areas in your routine.

Core strength can be improved through abdominal exercises such as crunches, leg raises or holding the plank position, however if you're not used to doing these types of movements or have any back or joint pain, I would recommend attending a Pilates class where you can get some support to do them safely.

For pelvic floor support, depending on how affected you are, you may be fine with some regular Kegel-type exercises, or you may need to seek out specialist help from a physio or pelvic floor expert.

Kegel exercises are designed to strengthen the muscles around your pelvis and bladder, and therefore help avoid leakage and incontinence.

However, a word of caution, it's easy to do them incorrectly and not only miss out on the benefits, but potentially make things worse. It's thought over a third of those attempting Kegels end up engaging their abdominal, buttock or inner thigh muscles instead of the pelvic floor muscles. So, take the time to get the basics right and if you are unsure, check in with an expert.

The good thing about Kegels is that once you have the hang of them, you can practise anywhere: waiting for a bus, waiting by a photocopier, riding in a lift. Anywhere where you have a few seconds to spare – squeeze in a Kegel!

How to do Kegel exercises properly;

- **Find the right muscles:** Start by identifying the muscles you need to target. The easiest way to do this is while you're urinating; try to stop the flow midstream. The muscles you engage to achieve this are your pelvic floor muscles. However, don't make a habit of starting and stopping your urine flow during urination, as it can lead to other issues.

- **Empty your bladder**: Before you begin your Kegel exercises, make sure your bladder is empty. This prevents any potential discomfort during the exercise.
- **Get comfortable:** Find a quiet, comfortable place to sit or lie down. You can choose to sit in a chair, on the floor or even lie on your back, but make sure your spine is straight.
- **Relax your body:** Start by taking a few deep breaths to relax your body, particularly your abdomen, thighs and buttocks. Tension in these areas can interfere with the effectiveness of Kegels.
- **Contract your pelvic floor muscles:** Squeeze as if you're trying to stop the flow of urine or prevent gas from escaping. You should feel a gentle lift and squeeze inside your pelvis.
- **Hold and release:** Hold the contraction for a count of three to five seconds, ensuring you continue to breathe normally during this time. Then, slowly release the contraction and relax your pelvic floor muscles for an equal duration.
- **Repeat:** Aim for 10 to 15 repetitions in one session. You can gradually increase the duration of the hold and the number of repetitions as your muscles get stronger.
- **Frequency:** get Kegel exercises into your daily routine. Consistency is key to seeing improvement.

Remember, it's essential not to overdo it. Avoid excessive squeezing or holding for too long, as this can strain the muscles. Also, do not perform Kegels while urinating, as it can disrupt your normal bladder function. If you have any concerns or questions, consider consulting a healthcare professional or a pelvic health specialist for personalised guidance.

Inspirational women: Linda Stephens

After suffering pelvic trauma with the birth of her third child, Linda used her women's health knowledge to heal without surgery. Seven years later though, she suffered a severe bladder prolapse while jumping on a trampoline with her kids.

When she discovered that prolapse susceptibility is due to the loss of oestrogen that happens during perimenopause, she went on a journey of education and discovery to heal herself again. She not only fully recovered, but now uses her knowledge to help others navigate the impact of hormonal changes.

As well as an experienced yoga teacher, Linda is a pelvic health expert and women's wellbeing champion, focusing her training and teaching on optimising women's long-term pelvic floor function so they have a better quality of life through menopause and beyond.

Linda's secret: Be in control of letting go of being in control. Acceptance is the key ingredient to change.

Listen to the full episode on the Happy Hormones podcast (ep. 94).

WALK MORE

Walking as a form of exercise is often snubbed by the fitness industry who try to persuade us to go big or go home! But if you're not able to do much cardio or weight training, walking on its own is hugely beneficial. Especially if you're navigating the world of menopausal hormones and feeling tired or stressed.

Few things have the power to restore quite like a brisk walk and a big deep gulp of fresh air. And the health benefits are many, from lowering your overall risk of chronic disease to helping you feel all is well with the world.

Health benefits of regular walking:

- **Heart health:** Walking reduces your risk of cardiovascular disease, high cholesterol and high blood pressure.
- **Brain function:** Walking increases circulation, therefore supplying your brain with more oxygen and nutrients. This can reduce brain fog, improve focus, concentration, memory and reduce the risk of dementia.
- **Diabetes risk:** Walking reduces the risk of type 2 diabetes by controlling blood sugar and insulin.
- **Bone health:** Low-impact weight bearing through walking can help prevent bone loss and osteoporosis.
- **Strengthens muscles:** Walking improves muscle tone and strength in your legs and back.
- **Supports immune system**: Walking helps to boost your immune cells.
- **Increases your vitamin D:** If you're outside you're more likely to make some vitamin D.
- **Reduces stress hormones:** Walking in nature helps to reduce cortisol.
- **Improves mental health:** Studies have shown that walking reduces low mood and depression.
- **Increases creativity and productivity:** I always get my best ideas when I'm out on a walk!
- **Longevity:** A recent study of 400,000 people found that just 15 minutes a day of moderate exercise (which includes brisk walking) can add up to three years to life expectancy. Even one ten-minute walk a week can prevent an early death by 15%!

Walking has other benefits beyond exercise. It's budget-friendly – no gym membership or pricey gear required, just get up and go. Plus, it's easy on your joints and bones, while helping to strengthen them. It's super convenient, too. Walk wherever you want, whenever you want.

How much do we need to walk?
Do we really need to walk the 10,000 steps that we are told is ideal? A recent analysis of over 200,000 people from 17 different

studies around the world showed a daily step count of around 4,000 can reduce the overall risk of mortality. Even just over 2,000 steps a day can reduce your risk of cardiovascular disease. However the overall conclusion was that the more you walk, the more the benefits, and that there didn't seem to be an upper limit.

Another study published in The Lancet found that for adults over 60, between 6,000 and 8,000 steps a day had the greatest effect in decreasing mortality, and for adults under 60 the range was 8,000–10,000 steps per day.

Tips to walk more:

- Invest in some good hiking boots for winter, comfortable trainers for summer and a waterproof jacket. Then there's no excuse not to get out, even if it's raining.
- Park your car further away so you can walk further. Every step counts.
- Get off the train or tube a few stops earlier, and walk the rest of the way (you can wear trainers and take your work shoes with you).
- Find a friend to walk with or join a local walking group.
- Take a stroll at lunchtime, or have walking meetings with colleagues.
- Meet your friend for a walk instead of sitting in a café.
- Get an app that records your steps if it helps to motivate you.
- Build walking into your daily routine.
- Get a dog – a dog is a great motivator to get out every day, but only if you can look after it and it's not going to add to your stress!
- Don't underestimate the power of 'just walking', adding in a few walks during the week could make a big difference to your health (and happiness!).

If you're new to walking or have been inactive for a while, begin with shorter walks and gradually increase the duration and intensity. Aim to get up to at least 30 minutes of brisk walking most days of the week. But check with your doctor if unsure.

NEAT

We know that exercise is crucial to overall health and wellbeing. But what if I told you that one of the most effective ways to boost your metabolism is to NOT exercise? I don't mean sit on the sofa all day. I'm talking about something called 'Non-Exercise Activity Thermogenesis' – luckily they decided to shorten it to NEAT!

So far, we've covered traditional forms of exercise that you're no doubt familiar with. NEAT refers to the energy expended in daily activities that aren't considered formal exercise, including everything you do between sitting, sleeping, eating and scheduled workouts.

In recent years, science is revealing that NEAT is an important way to boost your metabolism via your BMR (basal metabolic rate). This is the amount of energy your body burns through just staying alive (breathing, moving, heart beating, thinking, even fidgeting!). The higher your BMR, the more energy and calories you will burn off.

Your BMR will be individual to you, and depend on your age, fitness level, diet, lifestyle, genetics, weight, etc. NEAT can account for as little as 15% of energy expenditure in the very sedentary and up to 50% in very active individuals.

NEAT is not only good for burning more calories, it's also really good for our overall health. In one study, it was attributed to decreased risk of obesity, cardiovascular issues, metabolic syndrome and death.

The great news is that NEAT is accessible to nearly everyone, including those with disabilities, injuries, limited mobility, or those who simply dislike formal exercise.

Increasing your overall movement may require some habit changes, but even small adjustments can make a difference and boost your metabolism. Do what you can based on your abilities and preferences.

- **Sit less, stand more:** If you sit for your job, then try standing more often. It's not only going to increase your NEAT, it can reduce the harmful effects of sitting too much. No matter how many times a week you are exercising, it will not make up for a sedentary lifestyle the rest of the time. Try a standing desk, or just standing up when you're on the phone, or on Zoom, or when you're checking your emails.
- **Seated exercises:** If standing is not an option, you can still engage your muscles while seated. Try seated leg lifts, knees up, butt squeezes, calf raises, arm punches, or swap your chair for a stability ball to strengthen your core while you sit.
- **Take breaks:** When you're at your desk, set an alarm to move, either on your phone or on your computer. You can set it for every half hour, or hour, as a reminder to get up and move. Or if you're watching TV, get up during the ad breaks. You can go get a glass of water or do some simple stretches.
- **Walk:** As we've just seen, walking is one of the best ways to de-stress, improve your mood and stay active. Get a tracker so you can monitor your steps and get outside into nature as much as possible to get a mood boost.
- **Take the stairs:** Make a rule for yourself that you'll always opt for the stairs over escalators or lifts. Climbing stairs is amazing exercise – it's like a free gym! A recent study in the journal Atherosclerosis found that climbing more than five flights of stairs every day could reduce the risk of cardiovascular disease by 20%.

- **Stretch:** Incorporating some stretching into your daily routine not only helps keep you strong and flexible, but is also a great opportunity to move your body. I personally do some five-minute stretches every morning before I start work.
- **Active hobbies:** Doing something you enjoy that's also active counts towards your NEAT. Examples include gardening, cooking, fishing, dancing, DIY projects, photography, volunteer work.

Got a minute?

If you're super busy, don't have time to go to the gym or exercise for long periods of time, or you're low in energy or motivation, don't worry. Some research says you only need a few minutes a day to get benefits.

An Australian study found that just three or four one-minute sessions of vigorous activity daily, like brisk walking or running for the bus, could significantly reduce the risk of premature death, especially from heart disease, with up to a 40% decrease in overall mortality and an impressive 49% drop in cardiovascular-related deaths. Even a single two-minute burst of high-intensity exercise a day, totalling just 14 minutes a week, was associated with an 18% lower risk of all-cause mortality.

Just cutting sedentary time by as little as an hour a day, was linked to a 26% decrease in heart disease risk among women over five years, according to research from Harvard Medical School.

Lifting weights for as little as three seconds daily was shown to boost muscle strength, according to a study from Edith Cowan University. Three seconds!

So next time you catch yourself saying you don't have time for exercise, try simply committing to two minutes, and if you decide to continue beyond that, fantastic! If not, that's perfectly okay too. Even brief moments of movement offer remarkable benefits.

By embracing a well-rounded fitness routine that combines some or all of these activities, you can optimise your physical health, increase longevity and enjoy a higher quality of life for years to come.

SUMMARY

- Create your own mix of varied activities that you enjoy to reap the benefits of movement on your health and longevity.
- Sitting too much can shorten your life. Take regular breaks from sitting – use an app to remind you!
- Sweating helps to improve cardiovascular and lung function as well as support detoxification.
- Strength training helps retain muscles, improve bone health and improve metabolism.
- Stretching and mobility exercises improve flexibility and prevent injuries, as well as help you stay functional and independent.
- Look after your pelvic floor with Kegels or specialised yoga/physio.
- Walking offers numerous health benefits. Aim for as many steps as you can do in a day.
- General movement (NEAT) can boost your metabolism and improve general health.

CHAPTER 8:

B – BALANCE your hormones

All through a woman's life, maintaining hormonal balance can be a challenge. The natural fluctuations in hormones mixed in with life's inevitable ups and downs, means that hormone harmony is often impossible!

Once you're through the turbulent rapids of perimenopause, and into the calmer waters of post menopause, it should be easier. However, things may not be as smooth as you hoped. Many women continue to face significant stress in their lives, compounded by symptoms arising from lower sex hormone levels and other hormonal imbalances post menopause.

The bottom line is we still have to focus on hormone balance if we want to stay healthy and well as we get older.

In this section, I'm going to cover the Feisty Four hormones and how to keep them balanced, discuss the pros and limitations of HRT and how to stay real with the 80:20 rule.

YOUR FEISTY FOUR HORMONES

Cortisol

We know that too much cortisol over time can cause various health issues and accelerate ageing, so it's vitally important that we focus our attention on finding ways to manage our stress so that we can keep this one in balance.

The most effective ways to manage cortisol will be covered

under the Rest section next, where I'll talk about relaxation, sleep, breathwork and digital wellbeing.

In addition to these fundamental elements, there are some other ways to support your adrenal health:

- **Avoid food stressors:** Anything your body doesn't thrive on could be a source of stress. This can include the 'ageing foods' we have covered under Eat, nutrient deficiencies, food sensitivities, dehydration and food chemicals and additives.
- **Regulate your circadian rhythm:** Your sleep-wake cycle is really important in keeping your body in balance. Waking at consistent times, getting some daylight in the morning, winding down before bed, going to sleep at the same time each night will all help to keep this cycle working well.
- **The right balance of exercise:** Exercise can either help or hinder your cortisol levels, so getting the right type and amount of exercise for you is key. My general principle is that if you feel good on it, it's working. If you feel depleted and exhausted, it's maybe time to try something a bit more nourishing.
- **Minimise toxins:** Making sure your environment isn't adding to your stress levels is another vital tool to balancing cortisol. Jump to Chapter 12 Eliminate for more on this.
- **Manage emotional stress:** As we've seen, much of the time we spend in our fight-or-flight survival mode can be due to psychological and emotional stress. Whether it's from past trauma, life circumstances, relationships or other reasons, emotional stress raises our cortisol in the same way as if we are in physical danger. Jump to the Self section in Chapter 11 for more on how to deal with emotional stress, and Resources for links to professional support.

- **Supplements:** There are some key supplements that can help to support your adrenals. These include:

  - A good quality multivitamin (with active forms of B vitamins) – especially B5 and B6
  - Vitamin C
  - Magnesium (citrate or glycinate are well absorbed forms)
  - L-theanine
  - Herbal adaptogens – rhodiola, ashwagandha, holy basil, lemon balm, ginseng, Bacopa monnieri

- **Testing:** Testing my cortisol levels was key for me, as I didn't take it seriously until I saw it on paper! Jump to Chapter 13 for more information on testing.

Thyroid

We saw in Part 1 how important this little gland is for your health and wellbeing, and the significant impact it can have on your body if it's not working optimally. The range of symptoms can be vast, potentially affecting every part of your body and often overlapping with menopausal symptoms such as fatigue, weight gain, brain fog and mood issues.

Additionally, women over 40 are particularly susceptible to low levels of thyroid hormones, either through poor thyroid function or through the autoimmune condition known as Hashimoto's disease.

It's really important to identify whether you have a thyroid issue, especially since thyroid-related symptoms can mimic those of menopause.

Doctors in general are quite happy to test your thyroid, especially if you have symptoms. However standard testing is often inadequate to assess your thyroid health, for these reasons:

1. T3 is important. You will often only get two test results – your TSH and T4. If your TSH is too high, or your T4 too low, your doctor might prescribe you thyroid medication. If your levels are considered 'borderline' or 'normal' however, you will rarely get treatment, even if you have symptoms. The problem is that just testing TSH and T4 does not provide the whole picture. There is a complex thyroid pathway known as the H-P-T (hypothalamus-pituitary-thyroid) axis. TSH is your thyroid stimulating hormone – this is released from the pituitary gland in the brain to tell the thyroid gland how much T4 hormone to make. T4 is the inactive hormone that gets converted to T3, your active hormone. T3 is the one that does all the work, yet rarely gets included in standard testing.

For example, you might have normal TSH and T4 hormone levels, but low T3 levels, which suggests that your thyroid gland is producing enough hormones yet are not converting into the active T3 hormones. If this is the case, thyroid medication (which is T4) is not going to work. Instead you would need to support your natural conversion of T4 to T3 (through your diet, lifestyle or supplements), or look for medication that includes T3.

2. Thyroid antibodies are important. There are two main antibodies that can be picked up in standard blood tests: Thyroid Peroxidase Antibodies (TPOAb) and Thyroglobulin Antibodies (TgAb). Elevated levels of either can be associated with autoimmune thyroid conditions such as Hashimoto's thyroiditis and Graves' disease.

However, these are not always included in standard testing, and therefore the development of autoimmune conditions can be missed.

3. A very wide reference range. The 'normal' range for any given population is usually the range within which 95% of that population falls. That means that you could be 'normal' even though you are in the lowest 2.5% of the population. Unless you dip under this threshold, you won't get any treatment. Similar to adrenal function, thyroid disease is often only recognised and diagnosed as overt hyperthyroidism and overt hypothyroidism.

4. Inconsistent TSH ranges. There are many differing views on the optimal reference range of TSH, and it varies among laboratories. Many expert health practitioners like to see TSH levels below 2.5mlU/L for optimal health, corresponding with guidelines for pregnant women. However, in the UK, there is still no agreed consensus about the TSH cut-off value for treatment, with some labs having an upper limit of 10mlU/L.

If you suspect you may have a thyroid issue, make sure you ask your GP for all four thyroid measures: TSH, fT4, fT3 and TPO antibodies. If you can't get that, do consider seeking private support from a qualified health practitioner. See the section on Testing in Beyond Embrace for more info.

It might also be helpful to get some of your nutrient levels tested to make sure you are not deficient (especially iron, iodine, vitamin D and minerals).

Whether or not you are taking medication for hypothyroidism, there are lots of ways to support your thyroid naturally to improve your symptoms.

Natural ways to support your thyroid:

- **Eat enough protein:** Protein breaks down to amino acids, one of which is tyrosine, needed to make thyroid hormone. Protein also transports hormones around the body and helps to balance blood sugar.
- **Reduce sugar:** Too much insulin can impact your thyroid, so it's important to watch your intake of refined carbohydrates and sugar, and always try to eat protein and healthy fats with your food to slow the sugar release. Don't restrict your carbohydrates too much as this can also inhibit your metabolism and thyroid production.

- **Get your nutrients in:** Thyroid hormones need good nutrient intake to function well. These include:
  - Vitamin D (from the sun or supplements)
  - Vitamin A (e.g. liver, grass fed butter, animal products)
  - Iron (e.g. meat, poultry, fish, nuts, seeds, legumes, dried fruits, whole grains)
  - Selenium (e.g. Brazil nuts, sesame and sunflower seeds, brown rice, meat, fish, eggs)
  - Zinc (e.g. oysters, lamb, nuts, ginger, whole grains, sardines)
  - Iodine (e.g. fish and shellfish, sea vegetables, eggs, dairy, meat, sea salt)
  - Tyrosine (e.g. chicken, turkey, fish, avocado, seeds, nuts, dairy, whey protein)
  - Omega-3 fats (e.g. oily fish, flaxseeds, walnuts)
  - B vitamins (e.g. whole grains, oats, meat, dairy, green veg, nuts, seeds).
- **Try going gluten free:** Gluten has been linked with autoimmune thyroid disease (Hashimoto's) because the molecular composition of thyroid tissue is almost identical to that of gluten – which is potentially why your immune system attacks your thyroid as well as the gluten – a case of mistaken identity. Try going gluten free for four weeks to see if your symptoms improve.
- **Support your gut and liver:** An imbalance in gut flora can interfere with thyroid function and stimulate an autoimmune response against the thyroid gland, while some environmental toxins can interfere with thyroid function. Jump to Eliminate for more on gut and liver health.
- **Look after your adrenals:** Too much cortisol can suppress thyroid hormones. Follow my tips in the Rest section.
- **Move:** Activity can increase your metabolism, helping to get nutrients to your cells and endocrine glands, and helping to eliminate toxins. Check the Move section for more on this.

Insulin and blood sugar

As well as blood sugar swings which can drain your energy, store more fat, mess with your mood, give you constant cravings and fog up your brain, chronically high insulin is a huge stress on the body and a major health risk.

In Part 1, we discussed how insulin resistance becomes a greater risk as we reach menopause. The GOOD news is that you can lower your risk, and even reverse it, through your diet and lifestyle.

Diet: A blood-sugar balancing diet is key to managing insulin.

- Start your day with a protein/fat-based breakfast (or brunch if you're fasting).
- Include healthy fats and protein at each meal.
- Focus on slow carbs, e.g. vegetables, whole grains, quinoa, brown rice, buckwheat, millet.
- Limit refined carbs, sugar and alcohol.
- Try eating your veggies first, so that the fibre can take hold and slow down the sugar breakdown that's coming.
- A teaspoon or two of apple cider vinegar can help limit a blood sugar spike.
- Limit snacking, stick to two or three meals a day.
- If you do need to snack, make sure you add protein or fat to your carbs (e.g. apple with nuts or cheese, oatcake with hummus, celery with cream cheese, etc.).
- Try overnight fasting (12–16 hours), shown to improve insulin sensitivity.

Exercise: As we've seen, exercise is vital for your hormones. And it has a direct effect on how insulin works, increasing your cells' response to insulin (insulin sensitivity). That means insulin can get into your cells and drop off its glucose to make for energy. If you're not moving enough and insulin can't do its job very well, then you're at higher risk of obesity and diabetes.

Strength training is beneficial for preserving muscle mass, which plays a crucial role in glucose storage within the body.

Essentially, the more muscle mass you have, the greater capacity you have to store glucose. This leads to less insulin production, as the body becomes more efficient in managing glucose levels. A combination of HIIT and resistance training works well for this. And going for a walk for a few minutes after eating can make a big difference to your blood sugar regulation.

Stress management: Stress hormones exacerbate insulin resistance by promoting glucose release, interfering with insulin signalling, contributing to central obesity and creating inflammation. It's another vital reason to manage stress as we age.

Sleep: Your daily circadian rhythm is vital to healthy insulin management. Prioritise sleep, make sure you get some daylight when you wake up, and wind down at night (especially avoiding gadgets and artificial light) so that your body gets the right messages to make the right hormones (including serotonin and melatonin).

Jump to the next section Rest for tips on how to manage stress and improve your sleep.

Supplements: Certain nutrients can be helpful in managing your blood sugar and increasing insulin sensitivity:

- B vitamins (especially B3, B6 and biotin)
- Chromium
- Magnesium
- Zinc
- Alpha lipoic acid
- Curcumin
- Berberine
- Vitamin D

Testing: Start with your HbA1c levels. The doctor can test this for you. Other helpful tests might include your fasting insulin, or glucose tolerance tests.

Sex hormones

We know by now that declining sex hormones during and post menopause can cause all sorts of unwanted symptoms, as well as accelerate our ageing pathways.

While we don't require the same hormone levels we had in our 20s, it's helpful to have levels that effectively reduce symptoms and safeguard us against the potential health issues caused by low hormone levels.

The ideal hormone levels vary for each of us. Some women sail through menopause and feel fine in the years beyond, without any intervention. These are the women that might not understand what all the fuss is about (you've no doubt met one!). Whether it's their genes, diet or lifestyle (or a mix), it's very hard to know, but they are certainly in the minority.

Most of us will need some help, and that's where creating your own personalised toolkit can be a life saver. For some, HRT is their magic pill (more on that next). Others will prefer alternative solutions. Or you might be like me and adopt a combination of both. The important thing is that you are fully informed so that you can make the best choice for you and your unique body.

Regardless of whether you're on HRT or not, you will still need to support your health (and other hormones) through a balanced diet and lifestyle. Following the EMBRACE protocol will help you to achieve this, ensuring you have the best chance for a long and healthy life.

HRT (HORMONE REPLACEMENT THERAPY)

Unfortunately, with the huge increase in awareness recently around menopause, it has caused a big divide between those that believe HRT is the only answer and those that think the natural way to go is best. The last thing we need as women is to get dogmatic and start arguing among ourselves! Just when we are getting somewhere with women's health, it does make me sad.

What's most important is that every woman feels informed about her choices around what approach she wants to take. And she does what feels best for her. After all, that's what's been missing for all of us. Education and empowerment around what we can do for ourselves.

When it comes to HRT, I am not a medical doctor, but it's my job to know a lot about hormones and treatment options. And make sense of the latest research so that I can educate and empower women to make informed choices.

HRT certainly made the difference for me when my symptoms took a turn for the worse when I hit 50. I had my hormones tested and both my oestrogen and progesterone were on the floor. With my mum having osteoporosis, there was no way I was going to put myself at extra risk.

So, I did my research and chose to go onto body identical HRT in the form of transdermal gel and natural progesterone capsules. This combination has eliminated my night sweats and is helping to protect my bones, heart and brain.

I actually like to think of natural body identical HRT as just another supplement that can help us to rebalance. Just like vitamin D, which is actually a hormone too. And thyroxine which is given to replace low thyroid hormones.

Everyone now has access to body identical HRT on the NHS here in the UK. I'm not sure what's available in other countries, but body identical hormones are made from plants (mostly yams) and are molecularly identical to our human hormones oestradiol, progesterone and testosterone. There is no evidence to date of any associated increased risks to long-term health if taken correctly.

Oestrogen and testosterone are applied transdermally (e.g. patch, spray, gel or cream), meaning they go straight into the bloodstream once applied to the skin. This avoids having to be metabolised in the liver, therefore reducing risks of clots.

Micronised progesterone is the main form of natural progesterone available here in the UK at the time of writing this, and it comes in capsules. It is NOT the same as synthetic progestogens, found in combined patches, implants, birth control pills and the Mirena coil.

While doctors' knowledge and awareness are improving, I still hear many women are having issues accessing the right treatment or support. If your doctor is not supportive, ask for a menopause specialist or a referral to a menopause clinic if you have one near you. If that doesn't work, try a different doctor or practice. Or if you are able, there are many private doctors and clinics that can help. I have listed a few in the Resources section. Whatever you do, don't give up seeking the right support.

If you are taking HRT and it's not quite working for you, investigate these with your doctor:

- The format – is it body identical or synthetic?
- The application – try different ones to suit you (e.g. gel, patch, spray, pessary, cream)
- The hormones – is your combination of hormones working (e.g. oestrogen, progesterone, testosterone)?
- The dose – is it right for you?

You may need to experiment until you find the right combination for you and it may take a few attempts to get it right. Some doctors will prescribe higher unlicenced doses of oestrogen. If you are concerned about this, please get a second opinion or ask for further testing to ensure this is a safe option for you.

While there's no doubt that body identical HRT has many benefits, it is not a magic bullet. It is only going to help you if your sex hormones are out of balance or low. It is not going to help with any of your other hormones.

And it's not going to do much good if you drink too much alcohol, you're obese or you smoke. Studies show that these three things negate all the benefits of the hormones.

If you can't or don't want to take hormone replacement, we've covered many other tools that can help in this book, including natural herbal supplements and alternative therapies.

Whether or not you take HRT, the most important thing is that it's YOUR choice based on good information. Informed, personal choice is what every woman deserves. And you still need to adopt your version of the EMBRACE protocol to stay healthy as you age.

As women, we've been pretty much ruled by our hormones since we were teenagers, but once past menopause, hopefully you've got the measure of them finally – whichever path you've chosen that's right for you.

THE 80:20 RULE

A key part of a balanced approach to health and ageing is to be adaptable and flexible. It's not always possible to make healthy choices, and sometimes you just have to relax and enjoy life's pleasures without any guilt.

I wrote about the 80:20 rule in my first book, and it's just as relevant as we embrace this next chapter.

The 80:20 rule means that you prioritise healthy habits 80% of the time, while leaving a bit of room for indulgences in the remaining 20%.

For me, this has been a lifesaver over the years. While I'm passionate about nourishing my body with good nutrition, managing my stress on a daily basis, getting good sleep and moving my body as much as possible, sometimes it's just not achievable! In reality, life has other ideas, and it can be MORE stressful trying to fight it.

These days, I'm much more balanced than I used to be. I don't stress about eating gluten anymore. I'm lucky that it doesn't make me bloat or have any other symptoms. If it did, I'd definitely avoid it. But I love bread. I don't eat much, but when I fancy a piece, I opt for the best-quality sourdough I can find and I'm in heaven. And I enjoy the odd dessert or piece of cake without the guilt I used to feel (after years of yo-yo dieting!).

I still enjoy a glass of wine, but I know my limits and make a conscious effort to balance it with alcohol-free days during the week. I can also see a time not too far ahead that I might be happy to live without it.

If I don't manage my self-care on a daily basis, or I miss getting to the gym on the day I had planned, I'm not going to feel bad about that. If my 80:20 rule slips to 70:30 (or less), it's OK. When we beat ourselves up for not sticking to every habit we want to, then that just creates more stress.

The important thing is to have the right balance for you and where you are right now. Sometimes just getting out of bed every morning is enough.

SUMMARY

- Balance in our modern world can be hard to achieve, but if you can get your hormones working together more harmoniously, you'll be well on your way.
- If you focus on looking after your Feisty Four hormones, they are likely to look after you back, giving you more energy, focus, balance and vitality.
- HRT is an option that can help with menopause symptoms, however it's important to experiment with form, dose and combination, and remember it's not a miracle cure.
- Adopting the 80:20 rule for balance and flexibility around your health choices allows for enjoyment of life's pleasures while also nurturing overall wellness.

CHAPTER 9

R – REST enough

We saw in Part 1 how stress and cortisol make us age faster (and feel older). Excess cortisol breaks down muscle, promotes weight gain, suppresses the immune system and impairs memory, focus and mood. If left unchecked, it can lead to serious health conditions as we get older.

Therefore, a big part of the EMBRACE protocol to maximise your vitality and healthy ageing is proper rest and relaxation.

However, as a woman myself, and based on my experience running a women's health clinic for a decade, I'm going to take a punt that rest isn't one of your top skills (or priorities).

Rest and relaxation don't come easy to many of us here in the UK, but in other areas of the world, they have a better mindset. The Scandinavians for example have relaxation concepts that are embedded in their culture. For the Danes, it's 'hygge', creating cosy and comforting surroundings, while in Sweden they practise 'fika', the art of the coffee break for rest and connection. Similarly, the Dutch practise 'niksen' which literally means 'doing nothing' and allowing yourself time to unwind without any specific agenda.

In the Blue Zones, they have their own ways to reduce stress. The Okinawans have cultural traditions such as tea ceremonies, meditation, forest bathing and practising martial arts like Tai Chi and karate. In Ikaria, they take a nap in the afternoon. The Sardinians share food, wine and laughter with loved ones, while in Loma Linda, they pray. And in every Blue Zone region, they spend time outdoors, often gardening.

Getting more relaxation into your life may involve a shift in mindset, the development of healthy boundaries and a recognition that self-care is not selfish, but essential for wellbeing. Breaking free from deeply ingrained patterns and expectations may take time, but it is a vital step toward self-empowerment and overall health and happiness in this next phase of our lives.

SEVEN TYPES OF REST

Your version of rest may involve lying on the sofa watching Netflix, a lie-in at the weekend or a spa day once in a blue moon.

But according to Dr Saundra Dalton-Smith, "Many of us are suffering from a rest deficit, because we do not understand the power of rest … The result is a culture of high-achieving, high-producing, chronically tired, burned out individuals."

According to Saundra, sleep alone doesn't cut it. We need seven types of rest to switch off and feel fully restored.

Let's take a quick look at these:

1. **Physical:** Your body needs to shut down every day / night to recharge. Sleep is essentially your main passive physical rest time. And it's when the body repairs, regenerates and detoxes. Jump ahead for more on sleep, but adding in daytime naps and activities like restorative yoga and deep breathing can also help.

2. **Mental:** Your brain needs to switch off to minimise mental stress and fatigue. Take regular breaks and make some space in your life for things that bring you joy, let your mind wander or just to sit still and do nothing. Start slow with just five minutes sitting still, doing nothing. If that's unbearable, do some breathwork, listen to a mindful meditation or chilled music. Build up slowly as your body starts to thank you.

And remember to take your holidays from work – I'm astounded how many women tell me they don't always take their full holiday allowance. You don't need to spend money going away, just taking time out from work is so important.

3. **Sensory:** Our senses are bombarded on a daily basis: noise, light and technology are hard to avoid. This can frazzle our neurons. Time to reduce the overload. This can be as simple as turning off electronic devices, embracing silence, dimming the lights or spending time in nature. Be strict about work/home boundaries. If it's possible for you, make sure there's a cut-off between work and home. Find more tips on switching off from technology in Digital Wellbeing.

4. **Creative:** When fatigue sets in, it's really hard to be creative on demand. Creative rest can revitalise your creativity by engaging with the beauty around you, whether it's through art, nature or music. This type of rest can inspire new ideas, enhance problem-solving skills and bring joy.

5. **Emotional:** Emotional rest involves feeling and expressing emotions healthily, being honest about your feelings, seeking support and avoiding draining situations. This improves emotional intelligence, relationships and inner peace. Those who are givers, people pleasers or work in helping professions need this even more.

6. **Social:** Socialising can be exhausting, especially online (we're all Zoomed out!) and especially if you're an introvert. Balance social interactions by spending time with uplifting people and finding alone time, while limiting exposure to draining individuals.

7. **Spiritual:** Feeling disconnected from the world or your purpose can be draining. Sometimes just re-connecting

with our passion, purpose or just love of life is all we need to recalibrate. Try and find some quiet time to meditate or reflect (or pray if you have a religion). Start a journal or talk to someone close to you. Volunteer for a local cause or start your own movement if you want to have a purpose and make a difference.

Working out what type of rest you personally need is a good place to start.

If you're not getting seven to nine hours of sleep a night, start there. If you're snapping at everyone around you, perhaps it's emotional rest you need to prioritise. If your brain is foggy and you can't think straight, you're in need of some mental rest. You get the gist. Work out where your rest deficit is, and let's get Saundra's recommended 'rest revolution' underway.

Whatever you do, make your down time consistent and non-negotiable – schedule your rest time in your calendar and make it sacred.

THE POWER OF MEDITATION

There is extensive research on the power of meditation to enhance various aspects of health, including mood, energy levels, cognitive function, heart health and even libido.

Studies have shown that a regular mediation practice can reduce stress and anxiety, alleviate depression and increase positivity and emotional resilience.

Additionally, it enhances brain health by training the mind to be more disciplined and focused, thereby improving cognitive functions such as attention and concentration. Better sleep can be a by-product of that relaxation and stress reduction, as well as lower blood pressure and improved cardiovascular health.

Even more exciting is growing evidence that a regular meditation practice can positively alter your gene expression.

In 2014, researchers from the University of Wisconsin found that after a day of intensive meditation, participants showed reduced expression of inflammation-related genes. In another study, specific genes related to mitochondrial energy production, oxidative stress and cellular metabolism were upregulated after mediation practices.

Meditation can even increase activity of the enzyme telomerase, which keeps your telomeres healthy (those caps on your DNA) to slow down the ageing process.

It's not just health and longevity benefits that you get from meditation. A ten-year study of American executives found that meditation improved their productivity by 500%! And creativity explodes too.

Can you even imagine what that could do not just for the rest of your life, but also for the world? If every individual can find peace and harmony within themselves, the world would be a very different place.

If you haven't tried meditation before and would like to, there are many different types and styles, so do be persistent and find a course or practitioner that you love. I have just discovered sound bath sessions where you lie down and listen to waves of soothing, echoing sound from traditional gongs, Tibetan singing bowls or crystal bowls. The sounds and vibrations are incredibly relaxing.

My meditation journey

After learning about the power of meditation during my nutrition training in my mid 40s, I created a 'morning ritual' where I got up at 6am, did some yoga stretches, and then sat down to meditate for 20 minutes. I did this religiously for five years and loved the benefits I got from it.

However at some point in my early 50s, my need for sleep took over and I couldn't get up that early anymore. And just like that, my routine was broken. And so was my meditation practice.

I didn't really notice any adverse effects on my life until the end of 2022 as we were coming out of the pandemic. I was absolutely exhausted, and close to burnout. I had lost myself so much in work, that I had totally neglected my self-care.

I had to get back to some form of stillness. I knew I needed it, but I struggled for ages to find a way. My old meditations were not calling me, and I couldn't find an alternative that I could embrace as a new habit.

Then I discovered Dr Joe Dispenza, and after reading his books, I started listening to his meditations (he has plenty on YouTube if you want to check them out), and then attended his two-day retreat. It was an amazing life-changing experience, one I'd highly recommend if you're looking to improve your happiness and health.

I feel like I have rediscovered my joy and love of life. It was always there, I'd just let 'stuff' get in the way. And the best bit? I have learned how to access it whenever I want. It's truly such a gift.

If you'd like to know more about my experience at the retreat, check out my blog here: www.happyhormonesforlife.com/dr-joe-meditation

A word of caution: while most meditation practices are perfectly safe, a small proportion of individuals may experience negative psychological effects such as anxiety, depression and dissociation.

SLEEP

As we discussed earlier in Part 2, achieving quality sleep is a cornerstone of healthy ageing.

But fortunately it's not just about the hours you put in – it's also about how consistent you are with your sleep routine.

A recent study highlighted the significance of 'sleep regularity'. That means going to bed and waking up at the same time every day, with as few middle-of-the-night interruptions as possible. Surprisingly, the study found that sticking to a six-hour nightly sleep schedule consistently might actually lower your risk of early death, compared to getting a full eight hours but doing it in a really erratic way. Good news if you struggle to get a full eight hours of sleep a night regularly.

If you've already addressed the fundamentals of getting 'quality' sleep that I detailed in Part 2 (Sleep like a baby), let's dive a bit deeper into some more advanced sleep strategies that can help.

Chrononutrition: By synchronising your eating patterns with your body's natural rhythms (or chronotype), you can enhance metabolic health and support better sleep quality. This might mean experimenting with eating earlier vs later or having more consistent mealtimes.

Acupressure and reflexology: These practices involve applying pressure to specific points on the body or feet, aiming to alleviate tension, reduce stress and promote better sleep.

Progressive muscle relaxation (PMR): This is a deep relaxation technique that involves systematically tensing and relaxing muscle groups.

Yoga nidra: Often referred to as 'yogic sleep', this is a guided meditation practice that induces deep relaxation and promotes restful sleep by systematically relaxing the body and calming the mind.

Cognitive behavioural therapy for insomnia (CBT-I): CBT-I is a structured therapeutic approach to addressing insomnia, focusing on identifying and changing sleep-disruptive behaviours and thought patterns.

Light therapy: Exposure to specific wavelengths of light to regulate circadian rhythms can be particularly helpful for those with shift work, jet lag or seasonal affective disorder (SAD).

Essential oils: Oils like lavender and chamomile are known for their calming and sleep-inducing properties. You can use a diffuser, apply them topically to pulse points, add them to your bedding or a bath, or incorporate them into massages to promote muscle tension relief and induce a restful state before bedtime.

CBD oil: Short for cannabidiol, CBD has been touted as a miracle cure for virtually everything! But much of the research is around how it helps promote better sleep through interacting with the body's endocannabinoid system, which plays a role in regulating various physiological functions, including sleep-wake cycles. By modulating the activity of receptors in the brain and nervous system, CBD may help alleviate conditions like insomnia and anxiety that can disrupt sleep patterns, leading to improved sleep quality and duration.

Napping: If you suffer from less than six hours sleep a night, it's really helpful to get a nap in when you can to help your body catch up. A study published in the journal Sleep Medicine found that a 20-minute nap can significantly enhance alertness, energy and mood.

Bed temperature devices: Devices designed to monitor and regulate the temperature of your bed can stop you getting too hot at night. These include mattress pads, mattress toppers or standalone units that use water circulation or air ventilation to adjust the temperature of the bed surface.

Sleep tracking: Technology that monitors sleep patterns, heart rate variability and other physiological markers can provide valuable insights into sleep quality and help you make data-driven adjustments to your sleep routine.

Supplements: Supplements can be helpful, including:

- Magnesium (the calming mineral) – essential for relaxing nerves and muscles. Threonate is best for sleep.
- L theanine (found naturally in tea) – can improve both concentration and sleep.
- L glycine – amino acid known to help calm the body.
- Herbs: valerian, chamomile, passionflower, lemon balm, lavender, ashwagandha, ginseng.
- Adaptogenic mushrooms – e.g. reishi, lion's mane.
- 5 HTP – as the precursor to serotonin, this can help with mood, but also conversion to melatonin for better sleep.
- GABA – taken before bed can relax and calm.
- CBD oil – shown to improve sleep and reduce pain.
- Melatonin (only available on prescription) – low dose and extended release is the best form.

Progesterone: Natural progesterone (not synthetic progestogen) seems to help with sleep in several ways. First, it can calm the brain by boosting GABA, a neurotransmitter that reduces anxiety and promotes relaxation. It also helps regulate body temperature in the hypothalamus, making it easier to avoid night sweats and hot flashes that disrupt sleep.

Progesterone can also improve the structure of your sleep by increasing the deep, restorative phase and reducing the number of times you wake up at night. It's also anti-inflammatory so can ease pain and discomfort, making it easier to sleep peacefully.

Natural progesterone is known as bio or body identical progesterone and comes in capsules (micronised), or you can get creams in the private sector.

As always, please consult with your doctor or health practitioner before starting any new supplements or hormones, especially if you're on medication or have a health condition.

BREATHE

"The breath knows how to go deeper than the mind," Wim Hof.

Unless you live in a bubble, you won't have escaped the buzz about breathwork in recent years. If you practise yoga or Pilates, you'll know about the benefits, and of course 'Ice Man' Wim Hof has made his breathwork practice famous.

Despite its recent popularity, breathwork is far from a new phenomenon. In many cultures, it has been practised for centuries. These days, breathing has evolved into a thriving industry, with a plethora of courses, coaches and retreats promising transformative experiences.

But you might still be a bit sceptical. Surely breathing is something we all do automatically, the body knows how to breathe right?

Well, it used to, but apparently our modern world has made it much more difficult for us to breathe properly. And scientists are attributing poor breathing to many health-related issues, including cardiovascular disease, hypertension and poor immune function.

Why aren't we breathing properly? Several factors can have an impact. Stress often leads to shallow breathing, disrupting the natural rhythm of our breath. Prolonged periods of sitting, often accompanied by poor posture, can restrict our lung capacity and inhibit deep breathing. Pollution and the presence of airborne chemicals can irritate the respiratory system, encouraging shallow breathing as a protective response. And we are spending more and more time indoors with no access to fresh air, not enough ventilation, and that can hinder the intake of essential oxygen.

Breathing in properly enables us to get enough oxygen into our body, and that's really important for oxygenating our cells and delivering nutrients to them. Breathing out properly enables us to get rid of carbon dioxide, waste products and toxins. It's one of our main detoxification processes.

Essentially, when we don't breathe well, we are not getting these benefits. So, learning and practising breathwork techniques can really help improve our health.

Benefits of breathwork:

- **Stress and anxiety reduction:** Deep, controlled breathing activates the parasympathetic nervous system, promoting relaxation and reducing the production of stress hormones like cortisol.
- **Improved sleep:** Practising relaxation and mindfulness techniques through breathwork can ease insomnia and promote restful sleep.
- **Enhanced mental clarity:** Breathwork helps to oxygenate the brain, aiding cognitive function, memory and emotional stability.
- **Pain management:** Deep breathing can trigger the release of endorphins, which act as natural painkillers.
- **Digestive health:** Breathing exercises can promote relaxation in the digestive tract and reduce symptoms of conditions like irritable bowel syndrome (IBS).
- **Immune support:** Deep breathing can help to increase oxygen intake and promote a strong immune system.
- **Cardiovascular health:** Controlled breathing can help to reduce blood pressure, improve circulation and lower the risk of heart disease.
- **Enhanced lung capacity:** Regular breathwork exercises can improve lung capacity and respiratory function.
- **Detoxification:** Proper breathing helps to get rid of waste and toxins.

Nasal breathing vs mouth breathing
In his book *Breath: the new science of a lost art*, James Nestor argues that even with a healthy diet, regular exercise and adequate sleep, achieving optimal health is impossible without proper breathing techniques.

He explains the critical importance of nasal breathing as opposed to mouth breathing. Nasal breathing acts like a natural air filter, cleansing and moisturising incoming air, which can help stave off respiratory ailments and allergies. It's also a trigger for nitric oxide production, which widens blood vessels, aiding blood pressure control and heart health. Plus, it encourages diaphragmatic breathing, preventing the shallow breaths that often accompany stress and anxiety.

While nasal breathing is generally recommended, there are situations where mouth breathing may be necessary, such as during intense physical exertion or when experiencing nasal congestion.

If you tend to mouth breathe during sleep, you can try using medical tape or sleep strips to gently seal your lips while sleeping. This encourages nasal breathing and may improve sleep quality.

Breathwork is something easy, cheap and super effective. It's a no-brainer for your healthy ageing toolbox!

Simple techniques to improve breathing:

1. **Diaphragmatic breathing (abdominal breathing):**
    -   Sit or lie down in a comfortable position.
    -   Place one hand on your chest and the other on your abdomen.
    -   Inhale slowly through your nose, allowing your abdomen to rise while keeping your chest relatively still.
    -   Exhale slowly through your nose, feeling your abdomen fall.
    -   Focus on making your breaths deep and even.
    -   Practise for a few minutes each day to develop this habit.

2. **4-7-8 breathing:**
    -   Sit or lie down with your back straight.
    -   Close your eyes and take a deep breath in through your nose for a count of 4 seconds.

- Hold your breath for a count of 7 seconds.
- Exhale slowly through your nose for a count of 8 seconds.
- Repeat this cycle a few times. It's a calming technique that can reduce anxiety.

3. **Box breathing (square breathing):**
   - Sit comfortably and close your eyes.
   - Inhale through your nose for a count of 4 seconds.
   - Hold your breath for 4 seconds.
   - Exhale through your nose for 4 seconds.
   - Pause for 4 seconds before starting the next cycle.
   - This technique helps with focus and relaxation.

4. **Alternate nostril breathing (nadi shodhana):**
   - Sit comfortably with your back straight.
   - Use your right thumb to close your right nostril and your right ring finger or pinkie to close your left nostril.Close your eyes and take a deep breath in through your left nostril.
   - Close your left nostril and exhale through your right nostril.
   - Inhale through your right nostril.
   - Close your right nostril and exhale through your left nostril.
   - Continue this pattern for several cycles.
   - This technique helps balance energy and reduce stress.

There are lots of breathwork coaches, courses and free resources online if you need further guidance and motivation.

ACTIVATE YOUR VAGUS NERVE

The vagus nerve is the sensory superhighway that connects your brain to most of your vital organs, including the heart, lungs and gut. And its true potential health impacts are only just being discovered.

In medicine, research on the vagus nerve has mainly been focused on treating epilepsy, depression, blood pressure and even obesity. But new research is discovering its power to reduce inflammation by inhibiting inflammatory cytokines – and that could be game changing for future disease prevention and treatment.

Activating the vagus nerve (often described as 'vagal toning') can increase HRV (heart rate variability), switching on your parasympathetic (rest and digest) system. It can also reduce stress by controlling your heart rate and lowering your blood pressure.

An easy way to incorporate some vagal toning in your routine is to do your breathwork. By taking deep, slow breaths, you encourage the vagus nerve to kick in and promote relaxation. Another great trick is to sing or hum. Singing and humming naturally stimulate the vagus nerve, and crucially increase your nitric oxide production which helps dilate blood vessels and defend against infection.

Other strategies thought to help include gargling, massage, laughter, cold exposure (like ending your shower with a burst of cold water), gentle yoga and meditation. And there are some handy devices you can buy that give off vibrations when placed on your chest that are claimed to stimulate the vagus nerve (although there's no actual evidence to back this up just yet).

The secrets of the vagus nerve are only just being discovered, but tuning into it and giving it some love is a smart move for stress reduction and boosting your overall health.

DIGITAL WELLBEING

While technology undoubtedly helps us stay connected (it was a lifesaver during the pandemic), we saw in Part 1 how being constantly switched on can impact our mental and physical health, and ultimately make us feel more stressed and disconnected from the real world.

The challenge is to find a healthy balance between using technology for positive purposes and minimising any negative effects it may have on our mental health and wellbeing.

Here are some tips on improving your relationship with your devices:

- **Digital detox:** Set limits on the amount of time you spend on digital devices each day. Try designated no-tech periods – this could be during mealtimes, the first hour after waking up, the hour before bed or at weekends. Have a drawer where you can store phones when not in use.
- **Tech-free zones:** Establish certain areas in your home, such as the bedroom, where electronic devices are not allowed. Charge your phone downstairs, so you avoid the blue light interfering with your sleep, and you're not tempted to do any late-night scrolling.
- **Social media fasting:** Take regular breaks from social media and connect with people in real life. Arrange coffee, lunch or a walk with a friend (leave your phone at home or switch it off).
- **Practise mindfulness:** Take time to be present in the moment and engage with your surroundings. Mindfulness can help you manage stress and anxiety and improve overall wellbeing.
- **Use technology to your advantage:** There are apps that can help you manage screen time, and help you relax and sleep.
- **Be mindful of your posture:** Poor posture can lead to pain and discomfort, so make sure you're sitting or standing in a way that is comfortable and doesn't cause strain on your body.
- **Manage notifications:** Manage your notifications so that you're only receiving alerts that are necessary or important to you. Turn off notifications for apps that are not critical to your daily life. Leave WhatsApp or other groups that are not essential to you.

- **Social media sabbatical:** Take a break from social media platforms for a set period, such as a week or a month, to disconnect from the constant flow of information and updates.
- **Holidays without devices:** Go on a holiday or a short trip where you leave your devices behind, or at least limit their use only for emergencies.
- **Seek support:** If you're struggling with digital wellbeing, don't be afraid to seek support. Talk to friends or family members or consider seeking professional help from a therapist or counsellor.

Reducing your screen time in whatever way works for you will help you feel more present and connected as well as reducing stress, improving your sleep and brain health.

Inspirational women: Suzy Walker

In her 50s, Suzy went through a midlife reinvention, looking for a new kind of happiness. She left behind her prestigious job as editor of Psychologies magazine, got divorced, changed her name, lived on a canal boat for a year with her son, then sold it and went travelling in a campervan around the UK.

She finally settled in Northumberland, where she writes as a freelance journalist and is working on her third book about her year on the canal. As a keen storyteller and writer, she founded the Alnwick StoryFest, celebrating the power of stories through writing, films and photography.

You can find her on her Substack platform (called HeartLeap), where she writes regularly on how to find happiness and joy in a busy world.

Suzy's secret: Always find ways to be creative. Creativity gets you back into the flow of life.

Listen to the full episode on the Happy Hormones podcast (ep. 149)

SUMMARY

- Proper rest and self-care are not just important, they are essential and non-negotiable for managing modern-day stresses.
- Make time every day for relaxation, in whatever form that works for you.
- Resist the strong societal and cultural push to be busy and productive all the time and ditch any feelings of guilt attached to doing nothing or slowing down.
- Protect your time, energy, boundaries and space.
- Prioritise your sleep, not only to function better day to day but to improve your long-term health.
- Breathwork is a great tool to have in your stress management kit – practise daily.
- Activate your vagus nerve to switch on your parasympathetic nervous system.
- Manage your relationship with technology, make sure you are getting the benefits and minimising the negatives.
- If you really commit to this level of self-care, the rewards will be worth it; a sense of calm that you may not have felt since childhood (or ever).

CHAPTER 10:

A – ACTIVATE protective pathways

While the rest of the EMBRACE protocol lays the groundwork for thriving post menopause, here we'll explore innovative modalities that go beyond the basics.

From the science-backed benefits of heat and cold therapy, fasting and calorie restriction mimicking, to brain support, cellular health and carefully selected supplements, this section aims to proactively activate your specific healthy ageing pathways.

Again, this is not meant to overwhelm you and I'm certainly not suggesting you do it all. You can skip it entirely and focus on the basics if you want to. This is for your own exploration, if you feel called to.

CELLULAR HEALTH

Back in Chapter 3, we looked at the various biological pathways that affect our cellular health as we age. Following the EMBRACE protocol will help protect your cells, however here are some specific tips to support these pathways.

Autophagy: This is the body's cellular clean-up process. It helps to remove damaged cells and regenerate new ones, which is crucial for slowing down the ageing process. Intermittent fasting, low-carb diets, cold therapy and HIIT exercise can activate this cellular clean-up process. Supplements to promote autophagy include spermidine, resveratrol, berberine and curcumin.

mTOR: This is a protein that regulates cell growth, cell proliferation and cell survival. Regulation of mTor can be achieved through a mix of fasting (switching mTOR off) with consuming good-quality protein along with phytonutrients (switching mTOR on). Too much sugar or refined carbs can over-activate this pathway and increase the risk of cancer.

FOXO3: This 'longevity' gene plays a crucial role in cellular functions like DNA repair, stress resistance, apoptosis regulation and metabolism. Helpful FOXO3 activators include fasting, exercise, heat therapy, drinking green tea and supplements including vitamin D and omega-3 fats.

IGF-1: Dysregulation of IGF-1 signalling can increase the risk of insulin resistance and chronic disease. To optimise IGF-1 activity for longevity, focus on reducing sugar and carbs, regular exercise, weight management and healthy lifestyle habits while considering potential interventions such as fasting and natural supplements such as resveratrol, curcumin and green tea, among others covered in the Supplement section.

AMPK: This is an enzyme that plays a role in cellular energy homeostasis. Activating AMPK can improve metabolic health, enhance insulin sensitivity and help in weight management. Natural compounds like quercetin found in apples and onions can activate this energy-sensing enzyme.

Sirtuins: Sirtuins are proteins that are involved in cellular repair, metabolism and longevity. Sirtuin foods, often dubbed 'sirtfoods', include kale, berries, dark chocolate, onions, turmeric, green tea, apples, extra virgin olive oil, parsley, walnuts, soy, buckwheat, chilli. Resveratrol, found in red wine and grapes, is a popular sirtuin activator (although best to supplement rather than drink lots of red wine!). Exercise and fasting are known sirtuin promoters. Supplementing with NMN (a precursor to NAD+) can help to activate sirtuin activity.

Mitochondrial support: Almost everything in the EMBRACE protocol can help to support your mitochondria. Supplements such as coenzyme Q10, alpha-lipoic acid, d-ribose and acetyl-l-carnitine can be helpful additions. Also, certain compounds encourage the mitochondrial uncoupling process, which helps reduce harmful by-products. This process is of interest in longevity research because it could potentially lessen the damage associated with ageing and age-related diseases. These compounds include urolithinA, glutathione and melatonin.

Telomere support: Antioxidant-rich foods, exercise, stress reduction techniques like meditation, and adopting a positive attitude can support telomere length.

NRF2 pathway: Consuming antioxidant-rich foods such as berries, dark leafy greens and turmeric can activate this pathway. Sulforaphane found in cruciferous vegetables like broccoli is another potent activator of NRF2, as is EGCG found in green tea.

Anti-inflammatory and antioxidant pathways: Key drivers of inflammation and oxidation include a poor diet, excess stress, a sedentary lifestyle, poor sleep, environmental toxins, underlying infections and poor gut health. An anti-inflammatory and antioxidant rich diet and lifestyle as indicated here in the EMBRACE protocol can support these pathways.

Methylation: Following all the steps of the EMBRACE protocol will help with optimising methylation (including sleep, movement and relaxation), however focus on consuming adequate foods rich in methyl donors like folate, vitamin B12 and choline, while also supporting cofactors such as zinc and magnesium. Supplement with methylated forms of B vitamins and trimethylglycine (TMG) if required, but seek advice from a qualified practitioner first.

PROTECT YOUR BRAIN

As we discussed earlier in Parts 1 and 2, brain health and cognitive decline is a common worry for many women over 50. And I'd say it's one of the most scary too. We all know of someone with or caring for someone with dementia or Alzheimer's – and women are twice as likely to suffer from it as men.

But it's vital to remember that mental decline isn't an unavoidable part of getting older. There is so much we can do to protect our brains. A study by the Lancet Commission on Dementia in 2020 found that by taking preventive actions in our 20s, 30s, 40s and 50s, we might be able to 'prevent or delay' around 40% of dementia cases later in life.

Another study called the English Longitudinal Study of Ageing followed 12,280 midlife individuals for 15 years. They found that having a rich cognitive reserve – shaped by factors like education, mentally engaging jobs, staying active, enjoying hobbies and having a diverse social circle – was linked to a lower risk of developing dementia.

In Part 2 (Banish brain fog and forgetfulness), I discussed a range of strategies to look after your brain, from nourishing foods to movement and relaxation techniques.

While those fundamentals remain crucial, let's dive a bit deeper here into some more additional strategies that can help to further protect your brain and reduce your risk of conditions such as dementia and Alzheimer's.

Train your brain: Active learning is a vital way to keep your brain young. Learning something like a language, a new skill or musical instrument creates new neural pathways. Playing sudoku, doing crosswords and puzzles, and other brain-stimulating activities can help you keep your brain active and neurons firing. My mother-in-law is 82 and still as sharp as ever. She does her daily crossword, reads books and writes a new poem almost every week.

Sleep: I have covered sleep in several sections already, but it's getting another mention here as it's SO important for your brain! Sleep is the time when the brain has a deep clean – it washes away the accumulation of beta-amyloid and tau proteins, the harmful toxins linked to Alzheimer's disease. This nightly cleansing not only promotes memory consolidation but also acts as a protective barrier, guarding against the onset of Alzheimer's disease.

Take a brain break: When we're constantly entertained, through TV, screens, social media, podcasts and more, our brain doesn't get any switch-off time to replenish. Take some time to either do something physical, do some breathwork or a meditation, or just sit quietly and do nothing. Turns out watching paint dry might be dull, but it's actually giving your brain some much needed downtime!

Social connection: Spending quality time with friends and family isn't just enjoyable, it's also a scientifically supported way to boost brain health. Interacting with others is like brain gym. It necessitates thinking, reacting, making judgements, remembering details about people and even evaluating responses, all of which provide valuable mental exercise for the brain. Human connection, caring for others, love and physical affection increases oxytocin, which according to recent research is showing potential as a treatment for cognitive decline and dementia.

Get your ears tested: Hearing loss can increase the risk of chronic issues such as social isolation, depression, cognitive decline, dementia and even shorten your life. But studies show that regularly wearing a hearing aid can reduce the risk of early death by 24%, as the devices may boost mental health and cognition.

Breathwork: A study done in 2023 showed breathwork resulted in a decrease in amyloid peptides associated with Alzheimer's disease. Participants simply inhaled for a count of five, then exhaled for a count of five, for 20 minutes, twice a day, for four weeks.

Coherence: When the brain is in a state of coherence, it means that the electrical signals produced by neurons are working together in a synchronised and coordinated manner – a bit like all the musical instruments in an orchestra playing in perfect harmony. Coherence can be achieved through practices such as meditation, breathwork, mindfulness or neurofeedback training, and research shows it can have multiple benefits for brain health, cognitive function and mental wellbeing.

Movement, strength training and nature: All have extensive evidence that they benefit your brain, so make time to take a walk outside daily if you can, even if it's just a few minutes. And lift some weights.

Hand-eye coordination: Playing sports like tennis, table tennis, pickleball and badminton, along with playing video games, musical instruments and crafts, enhance cognitive function, promote neuroplasticity, improve fine motor skills, reduce stress, improve mood and potentially lower the risk of cognitive decline and neurodegenerative diseases.

Music: Whether it's listening to music, playing an instrument, singing along to our favourite track or joining a choir, music is a multi-sensory activity for our brain.

Boost your BDNF (brain-derived neurotrophic factor): BDNF is a protein that acts like fertiliser for your brain. It supports the survival of existing neurons and encourages the growth and differentiation of new neurons and synapses. But as we age, levels naturally decrease. We can boost BDNF through exercise (particularly strength training), eating a healthy diet with lots of vegetables, omega-3 fats and protein, brain stimulation, reducing stress, breathwork and sleep.

Check your homocysteine: Homocysteine is an amino acid produced during the methylation process, and elevated levels can increase oxidative stress, inflammation and vascular dysfunction in the brain, leading to an increased risk of brain shrinkage, cognitive decline, dementia and Alzheimer's disease.

You can lower homocysteine by getting enough methylated B vitamins and omega-3 fats. There are tests that measure your homocysteine levels with an easy finger prick if you're interested in brain health.

Brain supplements: In addition to a healthy and varied diet, there are key supplements that have been shown to support your brain. I cover these under Supplements at the end of this chapter, including my top five basics for women over 50.

HRT: Both oestrogen and progesterone delivered in body identical form have been shown to improve brain health. Oestrogen has been widely studied for its neuroprotective effects, showing benefits such as enhancing synaptic plasticity, increasing cerebral blood flow, reducing inflammation, and protecting against oxidative stress, all of which support learning, memory, and overall brain health. Progesterone has a protective effect on the brain and nervous system by increasing GABA, a calming neurotransmitter. Additionally, it has anti-inflammatory properties that can protect us against cognitive disorders.

Phytoestrogens: evidence shows that foods like soy and flaxseeds may improve brain health by enhancing cognitive function and offering neuroprotective effects. Soy isoflavones, such as genistein and daidzein, have been shown to improve verbal memory and protect against oxidative stress and inflammation. Additionally, phytoestrogens' ability to bind to oestrogen receptors and their antioxidant properties may help reduce the risk of cognitive decline and neurodegenerative diseases, particularly in postmenopausal women.

There's no miracle pill to prevent or cure dementia coming anytime soon, so focusing on a healthy lifestyle is our best bet.

Inspirational women: Susan Saunders

Another of my amazing podcast guests, Susan found herself at 36, with a toddler and newborn, having to care for her mum who had just been diagnosed with dementia. Having also witnessed her mum caring for her grandma with dementia, she decided to do as much as possible to break this pattern for her and her daughters.

She immersed herself into the science, co-creating The Age-Well Project platform and book, as well as qualifying as a dementia prevention coach with American neuroscientist Dr Dale Bredesen, author of The End of Alzheimer's.

She now coaches women over 50 to build consistent habits scientifically proven to reduce dementia risk and optimise brain health. She's the author of three books about healthy ageing. The most recent is The Power Decade: How to Thrive After Menopause.

Susan's secret: Being endlessly curious about the world and how it works. I'm always researching and asking questions. That extends to my health too!

Listen to the full episode on the Happy Hormones podcast (ep. 147)

FASTING

Many of the ageing pathways I've mentioned can be improved by periodic fasting. Fasting was a way of life for our ancestors, so our bodies are designed for it.

Fasting ticks all the boxes for healthy ageing. It activates autophagy, boosts mitochondrial function, reduces oxidative stress and inflammation, improves insulin sensitivity, activates sirtuins, contributes to DNA repair and stress response, while promoting cellular repair and regeneration. It also mimics calorie restriction (CR), which has long been studied for its longevity benefits.

However, despite the substantial evidence showing the benefits of fasting for healthy ageing and weight loss, and the many health experts advocating it as a lifestyle for all, it doesn't work for everyone and might even make some people feel worse.

This is particularly true for some postmenopausal women due to hormonal changes that affect metabolism, increased stress levels, naturally slower metabolic rates, and specific nutritional needs that might not be met during fasting. Additionally, fasting can lower energy levels, disrupt sleep, and affect individuals differently.

It's especially not recommended for those with thyroid conditions, adrenal fatigue, blood sugar issues, a history of eating disorders, low BMI, pregnant or breastfeeding women, people with chronic stress, or anyone needing consistent nutrient intake for medical reasons.

Having said all that, fasting can be a highly effective tool for many women. One of the easiest ways to fast in my experience is 'time restricted eating', where you do your fasting overnight (while you sleep) and eat all your food within a certain time of day – e.g. 10am to 6pm.

The 16:8 method is the one that most people adopt. The idea is you leave a 16-hour gap between dinner and breakfast or lunch – and do that three to five times a week. That might mean having dinner at 6pm, then not eating again until 10am.

However, this might look different in your life. You might have evening commitments, or work shifts. You can adapt it to fit your lifestyle.

If you're new to any kind of fasting and want to see if it can benefit you, it's wise to start gradually, say 12 hours, and increase the time period to one you're comfortable with. The longer you leave the time period, the more benefits you seem to get. If you can do a full 16 hours, research suggests you're more likely to benefit.

You can have liquids during your fast, but only water, herbal tea, black coffee or tea. Some fasting sites suggest you can have up to 50 calories without breaking your fast (e.g. a bit of milk with your coffee), but there's no evidence to back this up as yet.

Bear in mind this doesn't give you licence to eat whatever you want in your eating period! You still need to get your nutrients in, so make sure you're eating as healthily as possible. And don't do it if you feel unwell or have any unwanted symptoms as a result.

METABOLIC HEALTH

To avoid metabolic syndrome (as discussed in Part 1), we need strong metabolic health. This helps to reduce our risk of insulin resistance, impaired glucose metabolism and abnormal lipid profiles.

The EMBRACE protocol will help to support metabolic health, but if this is an area you need to focus on specifically, then embracing a ketogenic diet may be a key strategy for you.

The ketogenic diet, commonly known as 'keto', has been touted by some as the magic pill for weight loss, and by others as downright dangerous. So, it's not surprising that it generates a lot of confusion.

What is keto? A proper keto diet involves significantly restricting carbohydrates and replacing them with fat as the body's main source of energy. This triggers a process called 'ketosis', where in response to the limited availability of carbohydrates, the liver converts fat into molecules called ketones, which can be used as an alternative fuel source by the body and brain. This metabolic shift can lead to improvements in insulin sensitivity, blood sugar control and weight management.

While the keto diet can offer these metabolic health benefits, especially useful for those with type 2 diabetes, obesity or metabolic disorders, it also comes with certain risks and downsides. The most concerning risk for me is that a hardcore keto diet can result in potential deficiencies in essential nutrients like fibre, vitamins (such as vitamin C) and minerals (such as potassium and magnesium). Other risks include constipation, kidney stones, higher cholesterol and muscle loss.

If you've tried any type of keto diet before, you'll know that the main difficulty is that it's really hard to stick to long term. A more attainable way to get the benefits of a low-carb keto approach, without too much restriction or negative effects, is to adopt a more moderate keto approach. For me that means including more carbs in the form of vegetables – a sort of 'green keto' style. That way you're getting plenty of nutrients and fibre as well as keeping your blood sugar balanced and reducing insulin.

An even more extreme version of keto is the carnivore or caveman diet. This diet commonly features just meat, fish, dairy and eggs, so it's very restrictive and often impractical. While I would not advocate this type of diet for most women, I have seen good results in those with certain debilitating health conditions such as autoimmune, metabolic syndrome and other inflammatory diseases.

Whatever you decide, it's essential to approach these types of diets with utmost caution and consult a healthcare professional before embarking on them, particularly if you have underlying health conditions.

HEAT, COLD AND LIGHT THERAPY

Harnessing the power of cold, heat and light in your wellness routine can provide a range of advantages to support you and promote healthy ageing.

Heat

Heat therapy such as saunas, steam and hot baths, has been appreciated for centuries all over the world for its wellbeing benefits, including:

- **Detoxification:** Sweating helps to eliminate toxins through the lymphatic system.
- **Enhanced sleep and mood:** Heat exposure stimulates the body's thermoregulatory system, resulting in a subtle drop in body temperature that prepares you for a restful sleep.
- **Boost growth hormone:** Heat therapy has been associated with boosting growth hormone production, which plays a crucial role in tissue repair, joint health and the maintenance of skin and hair.
- **Support the immune system:** Regular sauna use supports the immune system, promoting overall wellness and resilience.
- **Stress relief:** Heat helps relax muscles, alleviate stress, reduce anxiety and enhance overall relaxation and mood.
- **Improved muscle mass:** Regular sauna use can slow the decline in muscle mass, a condition known as sarcopenia.
- **Promoting heart health:** Heat can be as beneficial as exercise for your heart! Heat causes blood vessels to dilate, improving circulation of oxygen and nutrients throughout the body and combining heat with exercise is even better, improving blood pressure and cholesterol levels. One study indicated that longer sauna sessions (20 minutes compared to 10 minutes) were associated with a 52% lower risk of heart disease.
- **Enhanced respiratory function:** The steam rising from hot springs or a steam room can help clear the respiratory system and open up airways. This can provide relief for individuals with respiratory conditions such as asthma, allergies or congestion.
- **Longevity:** Heat therapy switches on your longevity gene FOXO3. A study conducted in Finland discovered that individuals who used a sauna two to three times a week had a 24% lower risk of death. Those who used saunas almost every day experienced an impressive 40% reduction in mortality risk.

Heat therapy helps to increase the production of HSPs (heat shock proteins). These proteins help repair altered and damaged proteins, which are a hallmark of ageing. They also act as antioxidants and reduce glycation (those sticky proteins that cause inflammation).

Different forms of heat therapy:

- **Saunas** – including infrared, Himalayan salt, steam or traditional coal, wood burning, or electric saunas.
- **Hot stone therapy** – placing warmed stones on specific points of the body can promote relaxation, circulation and enhance overall wellbeing.
- **Heat wraps and pads** – targeted heat therapy for relieving muscle pain and stiffness.
- **Hot baths, hot tubs and Jacuzzis** – can relax and soothe the body.
- **Hot springs** – hot springs have long been recognised for their therapeutic properties and have been enjoyed by cultures worldwide for centuries.

Make sure to stay hydrated if you're using a sauna or a sauna product regularly.

If you don't have access to saunas or hot springs, there are various products available on the market, including infrared home saunas, lamps, sauna suits and blankets, among others. Make sure to choose reputable products from trusted sources.

Note: with certain medical conditions, such as heart disease, you should check with your GP before using a sauna.

Cold

Chilly moments might be more than just uncomfortable; they could be a secret weapon for healthy ageing. Just as that ice pack can stem inflammation when you injure yourself, short bursts of cold exposure can kickstart genes that help us live longer, boost the powerhouse mitochondria in our cells, and even dial down inflammation. But that's not all, they can also amp up your immune system, help you sleep better and even assist in burning fat.

When your core temperature drops, it triggers a cold shock response, which stimulates various processes to protect you. Blood vessels expand and contract, reducing the flow of blood to the skin where you will lose heat. Noradrenaline (a key stress hormone) is released, boosting performance of brain and muscle cells, improving memory, mood and focus. Endorphins are released, enhancing the feeling of wellbeing (many wild swimmers report feeling elated and glowing after a swim). Muscles contract to generate heat (e.g. shivering). Brown fat activates, stimulating fat burning and glucose breakdown to generate energy and speed up your metabolism.

The body produces cold shock proteins in response to cold exposure which help cells adapt to the challenging environmental conditions and maintain cellular homeostasis. If you expose yourself to the cold often, the body gets better at burning more energy and becomes more resilient to stress.

Ways to benefit from cold exposure:

- **Cold shower or bath:** This might be difficult at first (especially if you're a hot shower girl!), but try gradually decreasing the water temperature, allowing your body to adapt. Cold baths or showers can help with muscle recovery, improve circulation and boost alertness.
- **Ice bath:** If you're feeling braver, immerse yourself in a tub filled with cold water. Start with short durations and gradually increase the time as you become accustomed to the cold. Research suggests that the ideal temperature range for a cold plunge is between 10–15 degrees Celsius (50–60 degrees Fahrenheit).
- **Ice packs:** Applying ice packs or cold compresses to specific areas of your body, especially after intense workouts or to alleviate soreness or inflammation, can be particularly effective for targeting specific muscle groups or joints.

- **Wild swimming:** If you have access to open water or a cold-water pool, swimming in cold water can be an invigorating way to incorporate cold therapy into your exercise routine.
- **Cryotherapy:** This is where you step into a chamber filled with extremely cold air for a short duration. This method should be done under professional supervision.

A little chill can go a long way in firing up your body's natural longevity boosters. But be careful, do consult with a healthcare professional if you have any underlying medical conditions or concerns before incorporating cold therapy into your routine.

Inspirational women: Emma Simpson

After the tragic death of her brother as a young man, Emma found her voice diminishing as the colour seeped out of her world. She discovered wild swimming which helped her cope with her grief, and water became the medium within which she healed, and rediscovered adventure, deep connection and utter joy.

As well as discovering the therapeutic benefits of cold water, Emma has rediscovered her passion for storytelling and having completed her first book, she is currently authoring two more. Her debut, Breaking Waves, is about the primal powers of femininity and water, with stories gathered from women around the world that demonstrate the power of connection and humanity in an increasingly crazy society.

You can find and follow Emma on her Substack platform 'Lemon Soul – a space to gather and know that you are not alone' – and her website www.emmasimpsonauthor.com.

Emma's secret: Wisdom from my dad – when times are tough, just wait ten minutes and it will pass. If it doesn't, just wait another ten ...

Red light

Red light therapy is a relative newcomer in the wellness industry. It uses the power of infrared energy without heat (or very low levels) to rejuvenate your cells at the mitochondrial level. It operates by emitting specific red low-level wavelengths of light that penetrate about five millimetres below your skin's surface (a great thing to combine with heat-based infrared saunas which go deeper).

Evidence of the health benefits of red light therapy is growing. So far it's been shown to help with sleep and mood by influencing the circadian rhythm and melatonin production. It may boost growth hormone levels and support the immune system by promoting tissue repair, wound healing and reducing inflammation. Studies suggest it can also improve skin health by stimulating collagen production, reducing fine lines, wrinkles and age spots, while enhancing skin texture and elasticity.

Furthermore, there's potential benefits in dental health, aiding gum tissue repair, reducing inflammation and accelerating healing after dental procedures. It also shows promise in vaginal rejuvenation by enhancing blood circulation and addressing concerns such as dryness, stress urinary incontinence and vaginal laxity.

As well as treatments being offered in many spas and beauty salons, you can also get red light face masks, dental applications and discreet vaginal devices to use at home.

SUPPLEMENTS

One thing we can do to ensure we are getting the vitamins and minerals we need to age well is to take some key supplements.

I often get asked, 'but I'm eating a really healthy diet, do I still need to supplement?'

The answer is yes! In the years we've been testing women in

our clinic, it's clear that nutrient deficiencies are common. This can be for several reasons. You may not be getting everything you need in your diet. Additionally, food quality is not what it used to be, with produce grown in mineral-depleted soil or exposed to chemicals potentially lacking adequate nutrient levels.

Stress can also deplete essential nutrients required by the adrenals, such as magnesium, vitamin C and B vitamins. Limited sunlight exposure during winter months or among those with darker skin or who cover up, can lead to insufficient vitamin D levels. Poor gut health also affects nutrient absorption, even when consuming nutrient-rich foods. Lastly, just getting older increases nutrient requirements!

Therefore supplements can be really helpful to support your diet as you get older. But remember that supplements can't replace a nutritious diet and a healthy lifestyle. They really are 'supplemental' to these foundations, and to get maximum benefit from them it's advisable to work with a health practitioner who can create a personalised supplement protocol for you.

For some of our favourite brands that we use in our clinic, visit www.happyhormonesforlife.com/shop-now

Basics

These are my top five basics for general health and hormone balance for women over 50:

1. **Multivitamin/mineral:** I'm not talking about your average multi on sale in the supermarket – they are not going to contain the right forms or doses of many of the nutrients you need. Choose a brand that includes:
   - B vitamins in their active and methylated forms that are absorbable (e.g. vitamin B6 as pyridoxal-5-phosphate, B12 as methylcobalamin).
   - Vitamin A as retinol (not just beta-carotene) – this is the form that is most utilised by the body

- Key minerals: zinc, chromium, iron, magnesium, selenium, iodine.

2. **Vitamin D3 with K2:** We know the importance of supplementing with vitamin D (covered under Micronutrients), but it's helpful to include vitamin K2. While vitamin D helps your body absorb more calcium for bone health, vitamin K2 helps calcium get into the right places. K2 also works synergistically with vitamin D to support immune function and regulate inflammation. We don't get enough sun to make enough vitamin D year-round and K2 food sources are quite restricted, so we need to supplement with both, especially through the winter months. Aim for 2000–4000iu per day, depending on your levels and sun exposure.

3. **Vitamin C:** As well as fighting infection and immune support, vitamin C is a potent antioxidant, meaning that it prevents too much oxidative stress protecting our cells and our DNA from damage. It is needed for the production of collagen, the major component of skin, bone and connective tissue and it helps the adrenals to produce cortisol, so can get depleted when we're stressed. It's also key for protecting your brain cells from too much oxidation. Aim for 1000mg per day of the slow-release format, add more when you have a cold or infection.

4. **Magnesium:** Another common deficiency when tested, magnesium is so important, especially as we get older. It is responsible for over 300 different enzyme reactions in the body, including energy production, adrenal support, heart and bone health. It's your relaxation mineral, so great for stress and twitchy muscles, and can be helpful for pain. It's also another nutrient depleted by stress. It can be hard to get enough in the diet (e.g. leafy greens, nuts, seeds, veggies). The most absorbable supplement forms are magnesium citrate (tends to loosen the bowel, so good for constipation), glycinate, taurate, malate and threonate. Great to take before bed as it can help relax the body and aid sleep. Aim for 300-400mg per day.

5. **Omega-3 in the form of DHA/EPA:** Vital for brain function, heart health, skin, hormones and cell health. Unless you are eating oily fish at least three times a week, you are likely not getting enough omega-3 fats. These are called 'essential fats' for a reason. They are critical for the structure of your cell membranes and reducing inflammation. They play an important role in reducing the risk of arthritis, heart disease and brain and mood disorders. DHA supports brain cell membrane structure and fluidity essential for memory and learning, EPA reduces brain inflammation linked to neurodegenerative diseases and mood disorders. There are many fish oils out there, but it's really important to buy a good quality brand, with good levels of DHA and EPA. 1g–3g per day seems to be the sweet spot in studies.

These five are my absolute basics for postmenopausal women due to ageing, stress levels, poor diet / poor gut absorption and hormone imbalance.

But I can't stress enough that you must check with your doctor or health care provider before taking any new supplements if you're on any medication or have a health condition.

Menopause supplements

If you are not taking HRT, and struggling with symptoms such as hot flushes, brain fog, low energy, mood swings, etc., then adding in some herbal supplements can be really helpful. Plants and herbs have been used for centuries to support women's health. Here are some of the most researched:

- **Red clover:** One of the world's oldest agricultural herbal extract crops, red clover has very high levels of isoflavones (natural phytoestrogens) that help to mimic the action of oestrogen and can be used to help improve many menopausal symptoms.
- **Soy isoflavones:** I like to recommend soy in food form as a phytoestrogen (only organic and unprocessed), however many studies show that taking isoflavones derived from the soybean as a supplement can also be beneficial,

especially for reducing hot flushes and protecting against bone loss.

- **Black cohosh:** A North American perennial herb that has been used to treat gynaecological complaints for centuries, black cohosh is commonly used to help with menopausal symptoms such as hot flushes.
- **Dong quai:** One of the most commonly prescribed Chinese herbs for problems unique to women, dong quai has been traditionally known as 'a female tonic'.
- **Hops:** Recent studies have shown that hops may help women cope with hot flushes, sweating, restlessness and irritability.
- **Sage:** The sage plant has been shown to provide some real benefits for common menopausal symptoms.
- **Chasteberry:** Research shows that chasteberry (or vitex agnus castus) can increase LH (luteinizing hormone) and helps to inhibit the release of FSH (follicle-stimulating hormone), which can help to raise progesterone levels.
- **St John's wort:** Sometimes referred to as 'nature's antidepressant', studies have shown that taking St John's wort can provide a significant improvement in psychological and psychosomatic symptoms of menopause.
- **Maca:** Maca is a plant grown in Peru, and used for centuries for energy, stamina and hormone balance. The Peruvian nickname for it is 'nature's Viagra' due to its ability to help with stamina and libido!
- **Ashwagandha, rhodiola, Siberian ginseng, holy basil:** Have all been shown to help with various stress and anxiety symptoms.
- **Valerian, passionflower, lavender, chamomile:** These herbs have been shown to support sleep and relaxation.
- **Sea buckthorn, shatavari:** Sea buckthorn oil is rich in omega-7 and can help with vaginal dryness, while shatavari (or the 'female rejuvenator' in Ayurvedic medicine) is known to help with heat and dryness.

Research on herbal remedies can be mixed, and results are very dependent on you and your individual biochemistry, so it's advisable to seek out a qualified medical herbalist for your own personalised prescription (see Resources), especially if you are taking any medication (including HRT or the pill) or have a health condition.

Collagen supplements

Collagen is a type of protein that pretty much holds our bodies together. It's like the glue of our connective tissue, strengthening our skin, hair, tendons, nails, cartilage, teeth, muscles and bone, and even the lining of our gut and blood vessels.

When you eat protein (e.g. meat, fish, dairy, soy, eggs, pulses), the body makes collagen from the different amino acids from the food. But as we age (even from the age of 25), collagen production starts to decline. And during menopause, it plummets by around 30%. Studies show that oestrogen levels are correlated with its production, so when oestrogen starts to decline, so does collagen. And that can show up as more wrinkles, dry saggy skin, thinning hair, brittle nails and joint pain.

As well as obtaining collagen from dietary protein, it can really help to supplement. Do buy from a reputable brand as quality really does vary. Visit the recommendations page for my favourite brands: www.happyhormonesforlife.com/recommendations.

Ageing supplements

In the fast-evolving field of longevity research, this section reflects the latest findings available at the time of writing. While I strive to keep it as current as possible, please note that the most up-to-date information may have emerged since this publication.

In addition to the basic supplements, I normally recommend for women over 50, these are some nutrients that have shown potential in studies for general healthy ageing:

- **CoQ10:** Coenzyme Q10 plays a crucial role in cellular energy production and serves as a powerful antioxidant.
- **Glutathione or NAC (N-acetyl cysteine):** Glutathione is involved in numerous physiological processes, including immune function, DNA synthesis and repair, protein synthesis and regulation of cellular signalling pathways. It is often referred to as the 'master antioxidant' due to its central role in protecting cells from damage caused by free radicals, toxins and other environmental stressors. Take liposomal glutathione for better absorption, or its pre-cursor NAC, which is often cheaper and more bioavailable.
- **Alpha-lipoic acid** (ALA): A powerful antioxidant that can help neutralise harmful free radicals, reducing oxidative stress and inflammation. ALA has been studied for its potential in improving skin health, reducing the risk of age-related cognitive decline and supporting cardiovascular health.
- **Sulforaphane:** A phytonutrient found mainly in broccoli sprouts that can help to activate the Nrf2 pathway, leading to the upregulation of various cytoprotective genes, enhancing antioxidant defences, detoxification processes and anti-inflammatory responses.
- **Resveratrol:** Can trigger anti-ageing metabolic pathways, sirtuins, DNA repair and metabolism, AMPK, autophagy and mitochondrial function. Found naturally in red grapes (therefore red wine!) but not enough for therapeutic purposes.
- **Quercetin:** Can help combat oxidative stress and inflammation, as well as potential to improve heart health, support immune function and enhance cognitive function.
- **Curcumin:** Anti-inflammatory, anti-oxidative stress, curcumin has potential to support joint health, cognitive function and heart health. It may also have protective effects on the brain and nervous system.
- **Taurine:** A few studies have shown that taurine may enhance your body's antioxidant defences, potentially lowering the risk of conditions like diabetes, hypertension and cardiovascular disease.

- **Astaxanthin:** A potent antioxidant found in algae, astaxanthin has shown potential in longevity studies, combating oxidative stress, reducing inflammation and protecting cellular integrity.
- **Boswelia:** Has anti-inflammatory and antioxidant qualities, and can potentially support joint health.
- **Berberine:** Can help improve insulin sensitivity, regulate blood sugar and support heart health – crucial aspects of healthy ageing. Additionally, berberine appears to activate pathways associated with longevity and cellular wellbeing.
- **NMN:** NAD+ is a vital ingredient in our cells that helps with energy and repairs. As we age, we have much less of it, which can accelerate ageing. But we can boost our levels by taking a supplement containing NMN, which turns into NAD+ in our bodies.
- **UrolithinA:** A molecule that promotes mitogenesis, which is the formation of new mitochondria, and mitochondrial uncoupling which helps to limit age-related damage. It's found in foods like pomegranates, strawberries, raspberries and walnuts.
- **Spermidine:** A natural compound found in various foods, spermidine has shown potential for promoting longevity through enhancing autophagy, reducing inflammation, supporting cardiovascular health, providing neuroprotection and bolstering the immune system.
- **Crocin:** A natural pigment present in saffron, crocin has the potential to counteract cellular damage, reduce inflammation and support longevity while also helping to prevent cognitive decline.
- **Fisetin:** A naturally occurring compound in various fruits and vegetables, fisetin exhibits the ability to combat cellular damage, mitigate inflammation and promote longevity, all while potentially assisting in the prevention of cognitive decline.

Brain health supplements

As well as the basic top five supplements I have listed, which are all vital for brain health, these are nutrients that have also shown benefits:

- **Choline** (especially if you don't eat egg yolks): Supports the synthesis of acetylcholine, a neurotransmitter crucial for memory, learning and cognitive function. Alternatively you can supplement with lecithin.
- **Antioxidants:** To fight oxidative stress, including resveratrol, selenium, CoQ10, lutein, zeaxanthin.
- **5HTP:** Supports serotonin levels, which can help with mood regulation, reduce stress and potentially improve cognitive function and neuroprotection.
- **Vitamin B12** (methylcobalamin): Supports neurotransmitters, maintaining the integrity of the myelin sheath surrounding nerve cells, and helping to regulate homocysteine levels, which can reduce the risk of cognitive decline and support overall cognitive function. There's not enough in a multivitamin, and it's not always well absorbed, so sublingual lozenges in methylated form are best. Advisable to get tested before supplementing.
- **Creatine:** Women typically have lower body stores of creatine compared to men. Supplementing can enhance bone mineral density and has been shown to improve mood and cognition. Most women can experience benefits by taking a daily dose of 3 to 5 grams.
- **Nootropics:** See below.

Nootropics

Nootropics, often referred to as 'smart drugs', are a category of compounds, typically available in supplement form, designed to enhance cognitive performance, including memory, creativity, motivation and attention.

Some nootropics that have shown potential ageing benefits:

- **Ginseng:** Thought to support mood, reduce stress levels and combat brain fatigue.
- **Ginkgo biloba:** Known for its potential benefits for brain function and improved blood circulation.
- **Ashwagandha** has been shown to help reduce stress andanxiety.
- **L-theanine:** Found in tea and associated with increased creativity, relaxation and improved sleep.

- 248 -

- **Creatine:** Not only supports muscle function but has also demonstrated a positive impact on memory and reasoning skills.
- **Bacopa monnieri:** Known to enhance information processing, reaction times and memory.
- **Rhodiola rosea:** Helps the body cope with stress more effectively, as well as mood regulation and reduced mental fatigue.
- **Caffeine:** Surprisingly, your daily cup of tea or coffee falls under the nootropic category as it enhances alertness, attention and reaction time.
- **Mushrooms:** Several types of mushrooms have been classified as nootropics for their potential brain health benefits:
  - Chaga – rich in antioxidants and have been studied for their potential to support immune function and reduce inflammation.
  - Lion's mane – contains compounds that may stimulate the growth of brain cells and protect against neurodegenerative diseases.
  - Reishi – contain bioactive compounds such as triterpenes and polysaccharides that may have neuroprotective effects and support mental wellbeing.
  - Cordyceps – known for their adaptogenic properties, helping the body adapt to stress and promote overall vitality.

There are some prescription drugs that are showing promise in their use for extending lifespan, but they are still in the research phase, and their long-term effects and safety in healthy individuals are subjects of ongoing investigation.

Vegans

Whether your reasons for eating a vegan diet are ethical, environmental or health related, you do need to make sure that you're getting all the nutrients you need to be healthy and age well.

The nutrients you may need to supplement include vitamin A

as retinol, the active form, vitamin B12, vitamin D, iodine, iron, omega-3 essential fats as EPA and DHA, protein, choline and zinc.

If you're serious about implementing a supplement protocol to include some of these additional nutrients in your healthy ageing toolkit, it's really important to get support from a qualified health practitioner that can help create a personalised and tailored supplement protocol for you, based on your history, symptoms and goals.

And ALWAYS check with your doctor if you have a health condition or are taking any medications.

I've listed a LOT of different strategies here. PLEASE don't feel overwhelmed. This section is optional! I just want to show you how varied and exciting the longevity field is, and how we can take advantage of this new knowledge to benefit our own health as we age – IF that's something you're interested in exploring.

SUMMARY

- Switch on your protective pathways for cellular health.
- Prioritise and protect your brain.
- Adopt some form of fasting, whether it's just limiting snacking or your version of time restricted eating (but only if it feels good).
- Look after your metabolic health to reduce your risk of insulin resistance, obesity, heart disease and inflamm-aging.
- Try heat, cold or light therapy for all the health benefits they can offer.
- Supplements are an important part of your healthy ageing toolkit. Whether you take the basic five, or certain nutrients to help with specific issues, make sure you seek guidance from a health practitioner or medical professional.

CHAPTER 11:

C – **CONNECT deeply**

As a species, particularly in the developed world, we have become increasingly disconnected from each other, from nature and from ourselves. This disconnect touches every aspect of our lives, affecting how we relate to one another, how we interact with our environment, and even how we care for ourselves.

Most importantly it can hugely impact our physical and mental health. So if we want to make the most of our next chapter and live a happy healthy life, we need to make sure these vital connections are plugged in and thriving.

HUMAN

As humans, we are intrinsically wired for human connection. The need to belong is as basic a need as food, shelter and sleep, and it helps us live a longer, happier and healthier life.

As social creatures, we thrive on the warmth, affection and companionship that come from our interactions with others. From birth, we seek out social contact and are wired to respond positively to touch, eye contact and other forms of physical and emotional connection.

We have seen in Part 1 how loneliness and social isolation can affect our health and wellbeing, increasing our risk of depression, cognitive decline and a shorter life. We need interaction with others to thrive. Remember those Blue Zone centenarians? One of the common factors uniting them all was strong community and family relationships.

Strong social bonds can reduce stress, lower rates of depression and anxiety, and improve our overall quality of life. Daily contact with a social network (friends or family) has even been shown to significantly reduce the risk of dementia.

A detailed study at Harvard University looking at happiness and relationships of over 700 people spanning decades concluded that 'social fitness' was the most important factor for a happy life.

The researchers discovered that our relationships have a huge impact on our health. The stress from a sleepless night after an argument, or feelings of loneliness, have tangible physical effects on our bodies. On the flip side, happy emotions like the excitement of being in love, or the warmth of being truly understood, can positively influence our wellbeing.

Human connection is therefore as important for your health as your diet, exercise and all the other things we've been discussing. But looking at the studies and surveys in our post-pandemic society, our connection levels are not looking healthy. We're in a 'friends recession', with social fitness levels at an all-time low.

It's easy to feel like everyone else has their own *Friends*-style Central Perk coffee shop hangout or a *Cheers*-like local bar where everyone knows their name. Especially if you're on social media, it can feel like you're the only one missing out.

But find reassurance in recent data indicating that two-thirds of individuals are wanting to expand their social network, and that most factors contributing to the decline in friendships are situational, rather than personal (it's not you!). The reality is that circumstances and people change over time. Work commitments, families, health, relationship breakdowns, death, can all take people away from us.

With a little effort and focus however, you can create new connections and friendships that can help provide a vital piece in your healthy ageing toolkit. It does take some courage and ongoing effort, but the rewards are worth it.

So how can you start prioritising human connection in an ever-disconnected environment?

There are different levels of connection that you can develop depending on what might be missing for you:

Strangers
Even basic connections with strangers can decrease feelings of loneliness and isolation. Although you may never see them again, you feel better and you never know where it might lead. A study by psychologists in Canada sent participants into a bustling Starbucks with two different instructions: some were told to complete their visit as swiftly as possible, while others were asked to take a moment to talk with the cashier. The outcome showed that those who engaged in conversation left in a better mood and felt a greater sense of community and connection.

Here are some ways to increase interactions with strangers:

- Smile at strangers passing by.
- Start a conversation with someone on the train or at the bus stop, in the supermarket, coffee shop, gym or anywhere you might meet a stranger.
- . Introduce yourself to new neighbours, ask if they need anything.

Acquaintances
This group can be quite large as these are people you are not necessarily close to, but give you a feeling of belonging or community. This could include your neighbours, work colleagues, shared communities, friends of friends, distant relatives. They are important resources for when you need help or advice, or for sharing hobbies and interests (like cycling, gardening, reading, etc.).

This group helps increase our sense of belonging and community connection, and it may have some potential for deeper connections that you haven't yet identified.

Ways to develop this group:

- **Start an interest, join a club or movement,** e.g. book club, hiking, sports, hobby, charity, church, exercise class, shared cause. Activities with a level of interaction like this make it easier to engage with others as you have something in common. Make sure it's regular, not just a one-off. And be patient; it takes time to build real friendships.
- **Travel:** If you love to travel but can't find anyone to go with, go solo! Travelling alone is a great way to meet new people. Or book an organised trip with a group. These types of shared experiences are a great way to bond and make lasting friends.
- **Move offline:** If you know and regularly interact with someone you like online, try to meet up in the real world and see if it develops into a deeper friendship.
- **Volunteer:** If you've got some spare time and are looking to build connections, volunteering is not only good for the people you're helping, but also has a host of health benefits. Studies indicate that even if it's just a couple of hours a week, people who do voluntary work can feel less depressed, stay more active and even live longer.

If you are looking for deeper connections, have a look at who you might want to get closer to within this group. Who do you love bumping into? Who would you like to get to know better? Start with just one person and invite them for coffee, lunch or a shared activity. You may want to ask for practical help or advice they can provide. Ask them about themselves, be curious and listen – this engenders a deeper level of connection and meaningful conversations.

Inner circle

These are your closest relationships, usually close friends, family or partners who can provide safety, support, love, trust, joy and affection. It's where you can be vulnerable and your true self without judgement. Your inner circle is often quite small (mine is just a handful) – that's fine, as long as your connection needs are being met and you feel safe, secure and loved. This is where you need to spend the majority of your time and effort, either nurturing your current group or expanding it to meet your needs. Here are some ideas:

- **Prioritise your loved ones** – schedule time in your routine to spend quality time or connect with your inner circle, just like you would with exercise or self-care. This can be as simple as having meaningful conversations, going on dates with your partner, or enjoying shared hobbies and interests. Interestingly, even brief moments of connection can have a meaningful impact. A study revealed that a ten-minute phone call, repeated three times a week, significantly diminished feelings of loneliness within a fortnight.
- **Spend time with your grandchildren** – the Berlin Aging study found that helping out with childcare can reduce mortality rates by 37%!
- **Improve communication** – ask them how they are feeling, what they need. Open and honest communication is key.
- **Express appreciation and gratitude** for having them in your life. Small acts of kindness and expressions of gratitude can go a long way in strengthening the connection.
- **Emotional support** – be there for your loved ones during challenging times. Offer emotional support and understanding when they need it most.
- **Conflict resolution** – disagreements are normal in any relationship. Learn healthy ways to resolve conflicts, such as active listening, compromise and seeking common ground. Reach out to someone you've lost contact with due to a conflict (if you want that person in your life) – see if there's a way to resolve things (time can be a great forgiver).

- **Reconnect with old friends** – If you want to expand your inner circle, try reconnecting with a friend you used to be close to but may have distanced from. Or look at your acquaintance group for someone you'd like to develop a deeper connection with and build on that.

Bump up your oxytocin

Good relationships and connections give us a regular supply of oxytocin. This hormone is known generally as the 'LOVE' or bonding hormone and has all sorts of health benefits for us.

It's a hormone that is released in your brain (in your hypothalamus) with certain activities, most notably giving birth and breastfeeding. It's distributed by the pituitary gland to the rest of your brain where it can stimulate emotions of love, trust, connection, empathy, bonding and comfort. It also works with serotonin and dopamine, making these three a powerful trio of super happy hormones!

Oxytocin lowers stress hormones, protects the heart, calms gut inflammation, alleviates pain, promotes tissue regeneration, enhances sexual pleasure and conception, and may help with anxiety and depression. It's even being proposed as a treatment for Alzheimer's disease.

Human (and animal) connection and touch give us regular doses of oxytocin, so here are some strategies for increasing physical touch and oxytocin in your life (with or without an intimate partner):

- **Physical affection:** Increase opportunities for physical affection with family and friends, such as hugs, handholding, or a pat on the back.
- **Pet ownership:** Stroking and cuddling a pet can be soothing and provide a sense of companionship.
- **Massage:** Massage not only offers physical touch but also helps in reducing stress and improving overall wellbeing.
- **Participate in group activities:** Engaging in group activities or sports that involve safe, non-invasive

physical contact, such as dance classes or team sports, can be a way to experience positive social touch.

- **Mindful touch:** Mindful touch, such as self-massage or applying lotion with attention and care, can also be a form of soothing physical contact.
- **Orgasm:** Achieving orgasm (alone or with a partner) releases oxytocin and can have numerous health benefits, including stress relief, improved sleep quality, increased feelings of wellbeing, and the strengthening of pelvic floor muscles. It can also enhance emotional intimacy when part of a consensual and healthy sexual relationship.

Sex and physical intimacy

There is a common misconception that older people are neither sexually active nor interested in sex, however surveys show that older adults are indeed sexually active, although frequency does tend to decline with age.

A UK study in 2016 revealed how sexually active older women actually were. Two thirds of women in their 60s, a third of women aged 70–79, 14% of those over 80, and even 10% of those over 90 were still engaged in sexual activity.

Whether you want to have a healthy sex life or not (it's not for everyone), it's definitely more of a challenge as you get older.

Studies have shown 75% of women over 40 feel like their sex drive is decreasing, with 70% reporting dryness as an issue. Skip back to the section on Intimate Regions in Part 2 for all the symptoms of GSM that can affect our sexual activity.

As well as the physical issues we might face as we get older, psychological factors can play a huge role in low libido. Loss of body confidence, feeling hot and sweaty, or embarrassed by weight gain can make it more difficult to relax and get comfortable in the bedroom. If you're feeling low, anxious, irritable or flat, it's likely going to have an impact on your sex drive.

There may be underlying relationship issues between you and your partner, whether due to fluctuations in mood, life circumstances or other reasons. This can lead to a loss of intimacy or connection between you both, whether it's caused by your own challenges or those of your partner. Or you may be single and navigating the challenges of meeting someone new.

Ultimately, whether you're interested or not in maintaining sexual activity, there's no doubting it's good for you! The many health benefits include improved immune function, better cardiovascular health, reduced stress and anxiety, enhanced sleep quality and mood.

So, if you have a partner and are wanting to improve your sex life, here are some things to consider:

- **Talk to your partner:** Explain what's happening to your body during this stage (use my books if they help to explain things). If your partner can understand, they are more likely to be able to help and support you through it.
- **Prioritise your time together:** If you want to feel closer to your partner, prioritise your relationship. Make time in your diary to talk, go on a date, have sex or just be alone together.
- **Build trust:** Being vulnerable and allowing your partner to do the same builds trust. Share your fears, hopes and dreams, and create a safe space for your partner to do the same.
- **Relax:** Stress is a sure-fire passion killer! Make sure you take some time for yourself, whatever your commitments are (go back to section on Rest).
- **Look at your diet:** If you're not on HRT, phytoestrogens can help to replace oestrogen (soy, flaxseeds, red clover extract). Eat plenty of healthy fats (for sex hormones and lubrication), colourful veg, and avoid food stressors including alcohol.
- **Up your nitric oxide:** Nitric oxide helps dilate blood vessels and improve blood flow which can enhance

arousal and sexual response. You can increase nitric oxide levels through exercise, sunlight exposure, consuming nitrate-rich foods (e.g. green leafy veg, beets, celery), antioxidant-rich foods and stress management techniques.

- **Exercise:** Exercise stimulates circulation, blood flow and oxygen to all the right parts.
- **Switch to natural personal products:** Not only can many personal products irritate delicate areas, but they often contain hormone-disrupting chemicals like synthetic fragrances that are proven to mess with your hormones. Switch to natural products where possible.
- **Love your body:** Reframe your thoughts about your body (more on this in the Self section), be grateful for all the wonderful things it does for you.
- **Be more affectionate:** Physical affection, including hugging, kissing, cuddling and touching can help enhance emotional intimacy and trigger more arousal.
- **Surprise and spontaneity:** Keep the relationship fresh by surprising each other with gestures of affection or planned activities. Spontaneity can reignite the spark.
- **Supplements:** There are certain supplements I'd recommend to help with libido and dryness:
  - Omega-7 sea buckthorn oil – this can help with dryness.
  - Omega-3 EPA and DHA – healthy fats for good blood flow and hormonal balance.
  - A good multivitamin will give you the basic vitamins and minerals you need.
  - Maca is known as 'nature's Viagra'! The right forms off maca can help with energy, stamina and libido.
- **Natural lubricants:** Lubricants are helpful for dryness. Please avoid lubricants with chemicals in them that could irritate your skin. If they don't work then talk to your doctor about using localised oestrogen creams or pessaries, which are body-identical and low dose, so very safe.

- **Pelvic floor products:** If you have any pelvic floor weakness or incontinence, try yoga or Pilates, or specialised physiotherapy. There are also some devices you can buy that help to stimulate the right muscles.

- **Red light therapy:** There are products available that harness the healing powers of red light to strengthen the vaginal wall.
- **HRT:** Replacing hormones such as oestrogen, progesterone and testosterone can transform your libido and vaginal health.
- **Seek professional help:** If you're struggling to connect on an intimate level, consider couples therapy or counselling. A trained therapist can provide guidance and tools for improving your relationship.

Bad relationships

As well as cultivating good relationships, it's equally important to look at and deal with the bad ones. Not only does a negative relationship take a toll on your mental health, it also significantly affects you physically. Studies show that people in bad relationships or toxic friendships have a higher risk of heart issues compared to those in positive relationships.

Women experiencing high conflict in relationships often face elevated blood sugar levels, increased blood pressure and higher obesity rates. These relationships also put continuous stress on the body, keeping it in a constant state of alertness, leading to adrenaline overproduction, fatigue, weakened immune defences and potential organ damage.

I heard Reese Witherspoon recently refer to people as either 'radiators' or 'drains', and you should surround yourself with the former, those who radiate positivity, love and make you feel good.

Conflicts with others are inevitable, and there are things you can do to resolve them such as being more forgiving, not holding on to grudges, anger or resentment, and improving communication between you.

But if resolving them is not possible, it's important to let those relationships go and move on, for the sake of your mental and physical health, and ultimately your longevity.

NATURE

In a world where we're often surrounded by concrete and screens, getting back to nature can have significant benefits for our health, both mentally and physically.

There is so much evidence that spending time outdoors can decrease stress levels, lower blood pressure, improve our mood and even sharpen our minds. These benefits are especially valuable as we get older, helping us tackle some of the common issues that come with ageing and improving our overall quality of life.

Fortunately, there are many ways to tap into nature's benefits through the elements of air, light, water and earth.

Air
When we breathe in fresh air, the oxygen levels in our bloodstream increase. We need oxygen to sustain virtually every vital process in our bodies. It is the fundamental fuel for our cells, playing a critical role in energy production, brain function and overall physical health.

The health benefits of breathing fresh air extend beyond mere oxygenation. Fresh air, especially in natural environments like forests or parks, can have a substantial impact on our respiratory health. It helps to clear the lungs, reduce inflammation in the respiratory system and can even alleviate symptoms of allergies and asthma.

Fresh air helps improve our mood and reduce our stress levels, and spending time in oxygen-rich environments strengthens the immune system, making the body more resilient to illnesses.

To make the most of these benefits, it's important to get outside every day, whether it's a walk in the park, or simply relaxing in a garden. If this isn't possible for you, creating green spaces at home and ensuring proper ventilation can also help improve air quality indoors.

A regular breathwork practice can also help to increase your oxygen intake (jump back to Rest for more on this).

Light
As well as getting natural sunlight on our skin to make vitamin D, exposure to daylight is important for regulating our circadian rhythm, the internal clock that regulates various biological processes over a 24-hour cycle. When our eyes are exposed to natural light, especially in the morning (often called first light exposure), signals are sent to the brain's suprachiasmatic nucleus (SCN), the area responsible for controlling circadian rhythms. The SCN then initiates a cascade of hormonal and neural signals that help align our body's internal clock with the external environment.

Exposure to daylight in the morning helps switch off the production of melatonin, the hormone that induces sleep, making us feel more alert and awake. It also triggers the production of serotonin (our happy hormone) which enhances mood and cognitive performance. Regular exposure to daylight, particularly in the morning, can help combat seasonal affective disorder (SAD) and reduce the risk of depression.

As the day progresses and light exposure decreases, melatonin production increases, making us feel more drowsy and preparing the body for sleep. This natural ebb and flow of serotonin and melatonin is crucial for maintaining a healthy sleep wake pattern, which is essential for physical health, cognitive function and overall wellbeing.

Getting outside in the morning, either going for a walk, sitting in the garden or just opening a window or door to get some daylight on your face will help support this natural cycle. If this isn't available for you, light therapy using specialised lamps that mimic natural light can be beneficial.

Water

There's something about being in or near water that just feels good. Whether it's swimming in the sea, the sound of waves crashing on the shore, the peaceful stillness of a lake, or the rush of a river, water just calms you down.

Listening to ocean sounds has been shown to induce your parasympathetic nervous system, helping to reduce symptoms of anxiety and depression. Research has found that people who live near the coast report better mental health than those who live inland.

The soothing effect of water has been shown to boost creativity and cognitive function. Studies show that people who spend time near water score higher on tests of creativity and problem-solving ability.

It's thought that the negative ions in natural settings, particularly where water collides (e.g. breaking waves or rushing rivers), can benefit both physical and mental health. Recent studies show visiting waterfalls may improve lung function, immune response and reduce stress levels.

And of course, wild swimming has a host of benefits including being outside, exercising, community and not least the cold exposure.

Getting to the coast, or a local river, canal or lake on a regular basis is a great way to get these benefits. Much of my travel these days centres around some kind of water (we love canal boats as much as a beach holiday). But if that's not possible for you, there are many ways to enjoy the benefits of being around water. Consider a water feature, fountain or birdbath in your garden. The sound of flowing water can create a calming atmosphere. Or set up an aquarium in your home. Watching fish swim can be very relaxing, and a good way to add an element of water to your daily environment.

Inspirational women: Jo Moseley

In 2019, Jo, a single mum aged 54, became the first woman to paddleboard 162 miles coast to coast from Liverpool to Goole, picking up litter and raising money for charity.

It all started in the biscuit aisle at her local Tesco! Staring at the Hobnobs, she just started sobbing. Looking after two boys, helping both her parents through chemotherapy, and not sleeping, she was overwhelmed and exhausted. And unbeknownst to her, she was also going through perimenopause.

A friend suggested exercise might help. She started indoor rowing, then took her first paddleboard lesson. She was hooked! And it was the start of a new life of joy and purpose.

She's now the author of two books about SUP (stand-up paddleboarding), a speaker and host of her podcast, The Joy of SUP.

Jo's secret: Being outdoors – hiking, swimming or paddleboarding – has been hugely beneficial to my menopause. Find something that makes you feel good and which you can incorporate into your life. Start small, start today and start just as you are. You are worth it.

Listen to the full episode on the Happy Hormones podcast (ep. 110)

Earth

If you love the beach, you'll know how good it feels to kick off your shoes and feel the sand under your toes. There's a reason for that. The earth has a natural, negative electrical charge. When we have direct contact with it, we allow our bodies to absorb these electrons, which can help improve stress levels and boost our mood. It can also help neutralise free radicals and reduce inflammation.

You don't need to live near a beach to get this benefit. Walking barefoot on grass or soil will do it. Or get your hands dirty by doing some gardening. This might be why this activity is so popular, especially as we get older! It's certainly an activity that is shared among all of the Blue Zone centenarians.

Gardening has many other benefits. It's great exercise, contributing to improved mobility, strength and flexibility. Studies have showed that older adults who engage in gardening have better physical function and lower rates of disability compared to those who do not.

Other studies show that gardening helps lower your stress levels and improve your mood. Time spent in nature, along with some vitamin D from sunlight definitely helps. The interaction with plants can also encourage mindfulness and being in the present moment, which we know is beneficial for emotional health.

Gardening is also good for brain health. It often requires planning, problem-solving and attention to detail. It has been shown to reduce the risk of dementia in older adults.

I come from a long line of gardening fanatics in my family (on both sides), but I couldn't understand the appeal until just recently. For some reason, my gardening genes just suddenly kicked in and I'm now hooked. I can see now why so many people love it. Seeing nature do its miraculous work right before your eyes is awe-inspiring. My husband who has done all the gardening up to now is rolling his eyes (but is secretly delighted I'm finally appreciating it).

Even if gardening doesn't float your boat, you can still get lots of health benefits from being around plants in your home, garden, workspace or in nature.

Forest bathing, a concept which emerged in Japan in the 1980s, has gained global recognition for its health benefits. Research indicates that forest environments can increase the production and activity of natural killer (NK) cells, which help fight off infections and cancer. This boost is partly attributed to inhaling phytoncides, natural oils emitted by trees.

It's not just about getting outside, it's the quality of the experience that counts. Studies highlight that mindfulness plays a crucial role alongside simply being in nature. Engaging with nature through our senses – seeing, hearing, tasting, smelling and touching – unlocks its benefits (there's science behind hugging a tree!). Therefore, if you're distracted by your phone or other devices while you're outside, you might not get the full benefit.

There's no doubt that connecting and engaging with nature, through the air, daylight, water and earth can all be beneficial, so try to incorporate some of these tips into your lifestyle and see how it makes you feel.

Inspirational women: Lynva Russell

Lynva is my old boss and dear friend. When she retired from her role of CEO at a government think tank in London at 57 years old, she moved back to her home in Yorkshire, wondering what she was going to do with the rest of her life.

She knew she wanted to make a difference somehow, so set about investigating how she could help her local community of Holmfirth. She had always been passionate about the environment and saw an opportunity to help improve the quality of the River Holme as well as access to it for the community. What could have just been a litter-picking exercise was not enough for Lynva! She had much bigger plans, and soon enough River Holme Connections was born.

It is now a thriving charity, with over 100 volunteers and six staff, improving water quality, building footpaths, planting trees, creating new meadow fields and improving woodlands.

In 2023, Lynva was awarded the BEM (British Empire Medal) for services to the environment and West Yorkshire.

Lynva's secret: her 'can do' attitude, love for nature and community, teamwork and shared goals.

FOOD

We have never been more disconnected to food and eating than we are today. In the past, we knew where food was grown and how it got onto our plates – usually grown in the garden, in local fields or picked from a nearby tree, and always cooked at home. This close relationship with food didn't just make meals more healthy, it also meant we were more tuned in to what we were eating and how it affected our health.

Today, it's more about convenience. And understandably, in our busy lives, eating is another thing to fit into our jam-packed days – let alone the food shopping, preparing, cooking and clearing up!

In our bid to save time and effort, we are eating more processed foods and takeaways which are available at the click of a button. A global food supply means we no longer know where food is grown, what methods are used, or the journey it has been on to get to us. Online grocery shopping is another step that removes us from the source of our foods.

On top of that, we're not eating together as much anymore. Families used to gather around the table, sharing meals and conversations. Spending time in the kitchen as a kid with my mum, helping her chop veggies or peel potatoes, was really special to me. I remember the smell of her roast lamb with garlic like it was yesterday. Food creates memories that stay with you for a lifetime.

Nowadays, our fast-paced lifestyle often means that we all eat separately, grabbing fast food or microwavable meals on the go, eating mindlessly and without much thought about what we're consuming. It's so easy to eat on autopilot, scoffing down food because we're hungry, busy or comfort eating.

Convenience definitely helps us manage our busy lives, but in the process, this shift has undoubtedly contributed to health issues, both physically and mentally. Not only do we miss out on the nutrition and enjoyment that come from cooking or eating thoughtfully prepared dishes, but it can also put a strain on our digestive systems, and crucially we can miss out on those vital social connections that eating with others can provide.

Going back to those Blue Zone regions, the connection with their food is something that they all nurture and maintain. They eat mostly fresh, local and seasonal produce and have their meals in social situations, with family or friends. This undoubtedly helps them live a longer and happier life.

There are some ways that we can reconnect with our food in modern times:

- **Shop fresh:** Visit local farmers' markets or your local greengrocer when you can. Or sign up to an organic delivery service for fresh seasonal produce.
- **Cook from scratch:** Experiment with recipes, or get a recipe box delivery for inspiration. Try batch cooking at the weekend if you're short on time.
- **Eat mindfully:** Take the time to savour each bite and be present during meals. Chew thoroughly, wait between forkfuls, and avoid distractions like TV or gadgets. Mindful eating can help you tune into your body's hunger and fullness signals – it's been shown to help with weight loss and digestion.

- **Eat with others:** Make mealtime a communal event whenever possible. Sharing meals with family or friends can encourage connection and make eating a more enjoyable experience, even if it's just once a week.
- **Grow your own:** Even if it's just herbs on a windowsill or a small vegetable garden, growing your own food is a great way to connect with food and nature.

I realise this isn't always possible in our busy lives, but start small, do one of these things more and see how it affects you. I have found that the more I focus on this, my appreciation of food increases and so does the quality of my plate.

SPIRITUAL

When we talk about healthy ageing, engaging in some form of spirituality, whether through religion, personal beliefs or spiritual practices, can significantly contribute to health and longevity. In all of the Blue Zone regions where they are renowned for their longevity, people are tied together by some kind of spiritual faith or practice.

Spirituality is highly personal. It can be about being part of a religion, praying or going to a place of worship, but it doesn't have to be. For me, it's about feeling connected to something bigger, whether that's nature, the universe, source, your own inner wisdom or personal set of beliefs. It can be a knowing or trust that there is something operating at a higher or deeper level that is connecting us all.

Spirituality often provides a sense of purpose, community and emotional support, which are crucial factors in mental and physical wellbeing. Regular participation in spiritual activities such as prayer, meditation or attending religious services can reduce stress levels, lower blood pressure and enhance immune function. These practices promote a positive outlook on life, foster resilience against life's challenges and cultivate a deep sense of inner peace.

Research has shown that individuals with strong spiritual or religious beliefs tend to have lower rates of depression and anxiety and a higher likelihood of engaging in preventive health measures, ultimately contributing to a longer and healthier life.

Whatever spirituality means to you, finding ways to connect to whatever you believe in helps you to deal with stress, find community and maintain a positive mindset. All things we need to foster as we get older!

SELF

"The privilege of a lifetime is being who you are" – Joseph Campbell.

Self-connection is the deep, meaningful understanding and relationship we have with ourselves. This kind of connection is vital; it shapes how we engage with the world, make choices and sustain our relationships. Essentially, it's the foundation for our mental, emotional and physical wellbeing.

Self-connection begins with self-awareness – taking time to introspect, to really get to know who we are and what drives us. It means tuning into our thoughts, emotions, beliefs and perceptions. This is what drives our behaviours which ultimately shape our lives. The more awareness we have about ourselves, the more control we have over our thoughts, feelings and behaviours.

As we get older, self-awareness becomes increasingly important. It guides us through the inevitable changes and challenges of ageing, from physical transformations to shifts in our social roles. More than that, it builds resilience. By understanding our inner selves, we're better equipped to handle life's stresses and upheavals. It helps us remain adaptable, find new joys and keep a strong sense of purpose through the years.

With self-awareness comes self-acceptance, a crucial part of healthy ageing, especially for women. As we grow older, we see our bodies inevitably change. Embracing these changes is key to our emotional and mental wellbeing. It's about understanding that ageing isn't just a physical process but a reflection of our life experiences and growth.

When you find yourself wishing you were younger, would you really want to lose the experience and wisdom that you've gained throughout the years? Sure I'd like my younger looks back, but I wouldn't go back to my younger self for anything. Growing older is exactly that – it's self growth, and it's invaluable.

Beyond the physical changes, self-acceptance is also about recognising and adapting to our evolving needs. Maybe we swap spin class for yoga, stop dyeing our hair, or we start valuing a good night's sleep more than a night out. Whatever works for you, this kind of self-acceptance isn't just liberating; it actually makes us feel more confident, calm and content.

Self-connection and acceptance at this stage in life is empowering. It's a statement that we're comfortable in our skin and proud of our journey. It allows us to focus on what truly matters – our health, our happiness and the wisdom we've gained. This mindset can redefine the narrative around ageing, turning it into a period of life rich with experience, wisdom and a deep sense of inner peace and contentment.

Sharon Blackie writes of menopause in her book *Hagitude*, "During this period of intense physical change, it's also necessary to turn inwards, to embark upon the inner work of elderhood – the work of reimagining and shaping who we want to be in the world, of gaining new perspectives on life, of challenging and evolving our belief systems, of exploring our calling, of uncovering meaning, and ultimately finding healing for a lifetime's accumulation of wounds."

So where do we start? Things that nurture self-connection include mindfulness, meditation, journaling and engaging in hobbies or activities that we love. Knowing your values will help you have an inner sense of who you are and increase your self-esteem and worth. Your inner wisdom can be accessed at any time through being still, dialling in to silence and presence and listening to your body.

Let's look at several strategies to improve your self-connection, awareness and acceptance:

Prioritise your needs
We all have basic needs in life in order to feel OK. If we don't have these needs met, it can affect our energy, mood, drive, relationships, work and more. These basic needs include things like healthy food, enough water, movement and sleep. And there are usually others, and that will be personal to you.

For me personally, I know that if I don't have some form of affection in my life (hugs, physical touch), I feel out of sorts and lonely. So this is one of my basic needs to feel OK.

Other basic needs might include time in nature, music, prayer, friendships or alone time.

Have a think about what your needs are to feel OK. Journaling can be really helpful here. Make a list and audit each one. Once you start making sure your basic needs are met, you're going to have solid foundations to embrace this next chapter of your life.

Quieten your inner critics
We talk to ourselves in a way we'd never talk to anyone we loved! The inner critics in our head tell us we're not good enough, not worthy, not lovable, lazy, ugly, fat, old, the list of self-abuse goes on and on.

And we joke about the negative aspects of age all the time (just look at most birthday cards).

The problem is that your subconscious mind takes everything you say literally (and it certainly doesn't have a sense of humour!). It then relays what it hears to your body and cells to reflect exactly what you've said. So, the more you tell yourself you're old, ugly, fat, forgetful, irrelevant or useless, guess what? Your body responds by slowing down, withdrawing, living in fear and ageing faster.

The good news is that once we take notice of these voices, we can separate ourselves from them. The voices aren't who we are, they are like our safety guardians trying to protect us. So, if that's the case, we have control. And we have a choice. We can believe what they say, or we can choose not to.

We explored how these inner critics and limiting beliefs can affect our happiness and health in Part 1, where we talked about emotional stressors.

In Tara Mohr's book *Playing Big*, there's a fantastic chapter about limiting beliefs and inner critics. Here are her main tips on how to deal with them:

Identify your main inner critics. Here are some common ones:

- You're not good enough
- You're a fraud
- You're unlovable (nobody will like you)
- You're not worth it
- You don't fit in
- You'll never be successful

Tara's tips on managing your inner critics:

1. **Label and notice:** When you hear the inner critic talking, notice it and say to yourself 'oh, there's my inner critic'.
2. **Separate the 'I' from the inner critic:** Rather than 'I'm freaking out right now' you say 'my inner critic is freaking out right now'. It's just a voice within you, not YOU.
3. **Create characters for your inner critics:** Think of an image or name for it, so that you can see that it's not you.

4. **Understand its motives:** Ask it what it's trying to protect you from? Then reply, 'thanks so much but I've got this one covered.'
5. **Look for the humour:** It's usually ridiculous.
6. **Remove your inner critic:** Either stand or act like you're walking away. It's just me now, my IC has gone on a break.
7. **Turn the volume down:** Visualise a dial that you can turn down whenever you hear the voices.

My personal inner critics are 'You're unlovable' and 'You don't fit in'. I can pinpoint where these came from in my childhood. We moved around a lot as my dad was in the RAF, so I went to a lot of different schools. I was always the new girl, and it was hard to fit in and make friends. I've carried this throughout my life (it's hard-wired), but it's just a story I have made up about who I am, it's not true. And now I'm aware of the inner voices, I can distance myself from them and make different choices.

This new awareness in my 50s has brought a freedom that I hadn't expected. And I see this in other women post menopause. When you finally stop acting on those limiting beliefs and turn the dial down on the inner critics trying to protect you, you can start to focus on your own needs and desires. You can unapologetically and finally be yourself and not care about what anyone thinks. And that frees you up to go for your dreams, do things that bring you joy and fulfilment.

If you still feel like you're not fully being yourself, that you're continuing to wear a mask to please others, or you have suppressed a part of you or your feelings, Dr Gabor Mate suggests you ask yourself this question: *Where in your life are you not saying no?*

Healthy boundaries
Setting and maintaining healthy boundaries is crucial for maintaining our wellbeing and fostering healthy relationships. It's not just about saying 'no' more often (although that's important!), think about boundaries as the fences we put up around ourselves, defining where we end and others begin.

They're the guidelines we establish to protect our time, energy and emotions, ensuring that we prioritise our needs while respecting those of others.

Or as Brene Brown explains in a nutshell, "Boundaries are simply: what's okay and what's not okay."

By clearly communicating our boundaries and enforcing them with consistency, we create a supportive environment where we can thrive emotionally and maintain balance in our lives.

Here are five key strategies for setting healthy boundaries:

1. **Identify your limits:** Take time to reflect on your needs, values and personal space. Understand what makes you feel comfortable or uncomfortable in different situations, whether it's at work, in relationships or with family and friends.
2. **Be assertive:** Clearly communicate your boundaries in a calm and assertive manner.
3. **Practise saying no:** Learn to say no without feeling guilty or obligated to justify your decision. Remember that it's okay to prioritise your wellbeing and decline requests or invitations that don't align with your priorities or values.
4. **Set clear consequences:** Establish consequences for boundary violations and enforce them consistently.
5. **Seek support:** Surround yourself with supportive individuals who respect your boundaries and encourage your self-care efforts.

If you've never properly set boundaries before, you may find it challenging and may experience feelings of guilt or selfishness.

But as my friend Dr Joanna Martin (founder of One of Many) puts it: "Far from being selfish, setting clear boundaries is an act of great compassion. It means the people in our lives know where they stand. And it allows us to cultivate healthy, balanced relationships rather than simmering with suppressed rage at what we're having to put up with. And if it feels hard, remind yourself of this: you only need ten seconds of courage to set the principles that will save you huge amounts of resentment, conflict and energy in the long term. I've learned it's far better to cope with that little bit of awkwardness than the huge heap of resentment that builds up when you agree to things you don't want to do."

Here are Jo's three tips to create a boundary:

1. Acknowledge the request or situation, e.g. 'It's fine to ask for my help with …'
2. Simply and clearly state your boundary without justifying it, e.g. 'It's not OK with me that …'
3. Offer to try to find a solution together that doesn't cross your boundary (if appropriate) –'What do you need to give me what I need?'

Visualisation
Visualisation is a very powerful tool. Oprah Winfrey has spoken openly about her use of visualisation to achieve success. She credits it with helping her overcome a very difficult childhood, maintain focus and manifest her aspirations into reality.

It's a tool that's been used in sports for decades. They've even discovered that you can improve your strength just by thought alone, with no actual physical movement!

By imagining your desired outcomes with clarity and feeling, you trick your brain and body into believing they're happening right now. The brain then activates physical responses that make those visions real. Imagine how that could change your life?

Start by listing your goals. How do you want to feel or what do you want to achieve in the next phase of your life? The clearer and more detailed your goals are, the easier it will be to visualise them. The rest is practice and doing it consistently. Set aside a few minutes each day for this and see what starts to happen.

If you want to dig a bit deeper into visualisation, I highly recommend reading *Breaking the Habit of Being Yourself* by Dr Joe Dispenza. I mentioned before that I have rediscovered meditation through his teachings, and this book is where I started.

Do more stuff you love
Make sure you're doing something you love every day. Seeking out things that bring you joy is a natural antidote to stress.

It could be as simple as listening to your favourite music, reading a book, playing a sport, calling a friend, dancing around your kitchen, walking your dog or doing some gardening.

Being more creative boosts our happiness by giving us a sense of achievement, lowering stress, lifting our mood and putting us in a state of flow where we lose track of time and feel totally engaged and content. Try taking up a hobby you used to love doing but have lapsed. Did you used to paint or draw? Or play music? Or write stories?

Whatever it was for you, explore ways you can pick it up again. My brother was a really good artist in his younger days, but with work and a family just didn't have the time to do it. Now in midlife he has picked up his easel again and is loving it.

Or take up a new activity that you've always wanted to try, for example pottery, knitting, cooking, crafting, interior design, dance, playing a musical instrument, singing, writing or drama.

As we go from childhood to adulthood, the curiosity and imagination we had as kids can get buried under the need to be productive and achieve goals. Reconnecting with play can help us relax, boost our mood and bring some fun back into our lives. We can do this through spending time with our kids, playing sports, cards, board or video games, or organising game nights or themed parties with friends.

Laughter
Laughter is a key social connection and bonding tool. Humour and laughter have been used as medicine for centuries. It was even used as an anaesthetic before it was invented!

Laughter not only makes you feel good by releasing endorphins (you only have to watch a funny TV show to know that it feels good and lifts your spirits), but it also has other health benefits. It reduces stress hormones, works your muscles (ever had stomachache after a good giggle?), improves your lung function and circulation, improves digestion, heart health and immune function.

Children laugh more than 400 times a day, us adults less so (around 15 on average!). So, let's try to get more opportunities to laugh more:

- Watch a funny TV show or film, or go to a comedy show.
- Call a friend or someone you know that makes you laugh.
- Organise a night out with a good group of friends.
- Try laughter yoga (even forced laughter is beneficial!).

Shake up your routine

We've all heard the expression 'If you always do what you've always done, you'll always get what you've always got'.

As we get older it seems like the days can just blur into one. I know when I go on holiday for instance, the week will go relatively slowly, even though I'm really enjoying myself. Whereas when I'm at home, time wizzes by! Researchers have found that when we have new experiences, we dilate our sense of time in order to process the new information.

This concept ties in with Dr Tali Sharot's findings. A notable neuroscientist, she talks about the concept of 'habituation', how we get so used to our daily lives – our jobs, homes, even relationships – that the initial excitement starts to fade away. According to her research, our brains are wired to adapt and get comfortable with the familiar, and this can make our everyday experiences feel less thrilling over time. Just like a new relationship, it's exhilarating at first, then the thrill tends to fade over time as familiarity sets in.

The way to reignite that sense of joy and discovery, says Dr Sharot, is to introduce a bit of disruption and change. By switching up our environment, changing our regular routines, meeting new people, or even just imagining these changes, we can give our brain a sort of reboot. This helps us become more sensitive and aware of our surroundings again.

This approach isn't just about seeing the negatives that we might need to change; it's also about re-appreciating the positives that we've started to take for granted. Whether it's rediscovering the beauty in a well-known place from a fresh angle, finding renewed satisfaction in our work, or rekindling the joy in longstanding relationships, a little change can go a long way.

Stay present
Focussing on the present moment rather than dwelling on the past or fearing the future reduces stress, boosts mood and positivity. You can quickly bring yourself back to the present by taking a few moments to focus on your breath, noticing the sensation of each inhale and exhale.

Put your phone away and fully engage with what's going on around you and who you're with. Whether it's eating, walking, brushing your teeth or washing dishes, try doing it mindfully. Bring your full attention to the task at hand, noticing the details and sensations involved. If you're with someone, put your attention on to them, listen fully and be present – it's amazing what a difference this makes to how connected you feel to others.

Practise gratitude
Research shows that practising gratitude isn't just good for your mental wellbeing; it can also have a tangible impact on your physical health, including lower blood pressure, better blood sugar control and a stronger immune system. But let's not forget what it does for the brain – gratitude kicks off a biochemical dance that releases feel-good hormones like dopamine, serotonin and oxytocin. These neurochemicals not

only lift your mood but also reduce cortisol. So, when it comes to healthier ageing, gratitude isn't just a nicety; it's a full-on bio-hack that gives back, both emotionally and physically.

Start with just three things you're grateful for each day. It can be as small as having a comfortable bed to sleep in. Or a nice cup of coffee to start your day. Focusing on the good things in your life, however small, can make a big difference to your overall health and happiness.

Reframe your thoughts
We have already seen how your thoughts and inner voices can have unbelievable power to transform your life, for better or worse.

In Mo Gawdat's excellent book *Unstressable*, he says, "Stress isn't what happens to us. It's our response to what happens. And response is something we can choose."

If something frustrates or annoys you, those negative feelings will transmit to your body and cells. If you can change the negative thing, then do it. If you can't change it, you can at least change the way you think about it. Look for the silver lining in difficult situations and view challenges as learning opportunities. This doesn't negate the negative experience but adds a balanced perspective.

What may seem stressful and difficult to you, could be a totally different experience to someone else. Some people love public speaking, triggering positive endorphins and dopamine, while others will hate it and produce stress hormones.

My husband has been commuting into London for over 40 years, and I often ask him how he copes with the monotony and constant delays. He says he actually enjoys it, as he uses the time to listen to his favourite podcasts and it flies by. He reminds himself how lucky he is to have a job he loves, and time to himself every day on his commute.

How about rephrasing 'have to' with 'get to'. For instance, 'I get to go to work today and earn a living', 'I get to exercise today so I can be stronger', you get the drift!

For women, negative thoughts about how they look can be the most prominent. Here are some reframes to practise when you look in the mirror:

- When you hear a negative voice in your head about ageing or a certain part of your body, turn it into a positive and celebrate it instead.
- When you see a wobbly belly, think wow, that belly has brought a child into the world or that belly is keeping some spare energy in case I need it someday.
- If you see wrinkles, look at them as 'character' or 'laughter' lines, each one telling a story about your life.
- If you're grieving over the loss of your youth, body shape or younger self, remember that it's not loss, it's change. You're a different version of yourself that's more wise, experienced and resilient. Celebrate that and use it to embrace the rest of your life with positivity.

Practise saying one or more of these affirmations out loud – even if you don't believe them at first, the more you repeat them, you will start to feel more positive about yourself. And don't forget your subconscious mind believes what you tell it, so exaggeration is good!

- My body is a truly beautiful reflection of my life's journey.
- I am grateful to my body for the amazing strength and wisdom it carries.
- My body's changes are a natural and beautiful part of ageing.
- I honour my body as a remarkable vessel that carries me through life.
- Ageing is a huge gift and privilege many don't get to experience, and I'm very grateful for that.
- Every day, I'm looking and feeling so much younger than my years.

If you want a more structured approach (and in the UK you can often get a free referral), you may want to explore cognitive behavioural therapy (CBT). CBT is a psychotherapy approach that focuses on identifying and changing negative thought patterns and behaviours to improve mental health and wellbeing. It emphasises the connection between thoughts, feelings and behaviours, aiming to help you develop coping strategies, challenge unhelpful beliefs and learn practical skills to manage challenges effectively.

Inspirational women: Caroline Ferguson

My dear friend Caroline is a psychotherapy-trained mindset coach who helps women to challenge and change old beliefs, emotions and habits that are getting in the way, and gives them crucial skills for meeting their goals and creating a more meaningful life.

She had a profound realisation about her body that completely transformed her approach to self-care, which previously was rooted in negativity and self-hate. It was this: "My body is not a bunch of bits I don't like. It's my miraculous home for life – and I can't move out. It's up to me to make it the best home it can be."

And talking of home, Caroline decided in her 50s to sell up and embark on a new adventure, house and pet sitting all over the UK. Four years later, she's still 'homeless' and she's never been happier.

Caroline's secret: Recognise that self-awareness is the no. 1 life skill you can have. The more you build it, the greater your chances of peace, fulfilment and joy.

Listen to the full episode on the Happy Hormones podcast (ep. 133)

Implementing these strategies requires practice and patience. It's important to remember that it's normal to experience negative thoughts and emotions, and it won't be possible to eliminate them completely but the more positivity and appreciation you can adopt, the better your body will respond.

You may also need to deal with past trauma, emotions, limiting beliefs or low self-esteem. This might involve seeking a coach or therapist as you may need to dig deeper than you're able to do on your own.

Purpose, legacy and contribution

Several studies have shown a correlation between having a sense of meaning, purpose and direction with a longer life. We know from the Blue Zone research that purpose is one of the common elements in the centenarians studied. In Nicoya, Costa Rica, they call it their *'plan de vida'* or 'life plan' and in Okinawa, Japan, it's known as *'ikigai'* or 'reason for living'.

This can be even more important once you retire. Many retirees report feeling lost, bored or discarded by society. Finding a new purpose can be the difference between slowly degenerating towards the end of your life or thriving during these years with renewed vigour and fulfilment.

You might think having a purpose in life means somehow having to change the world in some way – that it's a big thing. And that can feel exhausting, especially when we're already exhausted and overwhelmed!

But a purpose is whatever lights you up or makes you feel fulfilled. It can be as simple as looking after your grandchildren, tending your garden, creating music, painting or drawing, writing a book, poems or stories, volunteering for a local cause or running a book club. Or you may want to start a new business or project. If you've got a grand purpose, great, but it doesn't have to be so big that you don't feel valuable or able to contribute to others.

Equally, your purpose doesn't have to be your career or main source of income. If your job or finances can support your purpose, that's just as good.

Engaging in legacy work and contribution can profoundly enhance your sense of purpose as you get older. Legacy work involves activities that allow you to reflect on your life experiences, share your wisdom and create meaningful contributions that can be passed on to future generations. This might mean writing your memoirs, mentoring younger people, volunteering or creating art. Additionally, contributing to charitable causes, whether through volunteer work or donations, can be incredibly fulfilling.

Contributing to others in this way not only enriches the lives of those who receive your wisdom and support, but also provides you with a strong sense of belonging and continued relevance. This increased meaning and engagement can lead to improved mental health, reduced feelings of isolation and a more positive outlook on ageing.

Take some time to think about what you want from your life and how you can contribute your wisdom and experience to others. What are you going to do with your possible 30–50 years ahead of you? If you don't know the answer to this question, don't worry, keep asking and your vision will develop over time. Meditation is a great tool for this, to quieten the mind and listen to your inner wisdom.

Vishen Lakhiani from Mindvalley, suggests asking yourself three questions:

1. What experiences do you want to have? What sort of things bring you joy? Do you want to travel? Do you want to meet someone special? What things when you think about them make you smile? How can you design your life to include more things that you love?

2. How am I going to grow? Humans gain fulfilment from personal growth. Do you want to learn something new? A new language, skill or tool?

3. How can I give back to the world? Whether it's volunteering, giving or working for a charity, teaching or mentoring people or creating something that makes a difference in the world, contribution of some kind is a vital part of your healthy ageing toolkit.

Most of all, this is the time to identify and celebrate your uniqueness. There never has been and never will be another YOU. You don't have to conform any more. You are free to be yourself, and to live life your way.

You may not feel you have enough money, time or energy for this right now. But stay with it. Keep your vision alive and do small things to move towards it. Keep journaling and meditating until you get the answers and see the opportunities.

Finding your purpose may mean you need to be brave. You may have to step out of your comfort zone to explore new things and there may be some disruption of the status quo in the process. And you may have to suffer the discomfort of uncertainty. But if we can sit with it for a while, learn to accept the fear of the unknown, and be open to what shows up, we may reap the rewards on the other side – more happiness, meaning, calm, fulfilment and peace.

Visualising your goals as if they've already been achieved can programme your subconscious mind for success. This mental rehearsal prepares your conscious mind to take proactive steps, turning your aspirations into tangible outcomes. This approach is grounded in psychology and can be an effective tool in achieving your goals.

Inspirational women: Karen Arthur

Karen is a grandmother in her early 60s, who refuses to become invisible post menopause!

Depression and anxiety hit her in her early 50s as a teacher and she had no idea it could have anything to do with menopause. Leaving her career, therapy and expressing her creativity through fashion were her breakthroughs. She recognised that other women were suffering too but she saw no one from the Black community amplified in the media. It felt like her experience didn't exist.

Lockdown and the global tragedy of George Floyd's murder galvanised Karen into reaching out to a wider audience. She started Menopause Whilst Black, the podcast to address glaring diversity issues within the menopause space. With her ground-shifting podcast, the first in the UK, she remains committed to giving voice to menopause stories of Black people experiencing menopause primarily based in the UK.

Karen's secret is no secret. Moving her body and getting outside – walking, swimming, running, resistance training and most recently, burlesque dancing! As long as it makes her feel good, she'll most likely give it a go.

Listen to the full episode on the Happy Hormones podcast (ep. 69)

SUMMARY

- Modern life can make it challenging to stay connected to others, to nature, to our food and to ourselves. Do everything you can to improve these connections.
- Human connection is as vital a need as food and shelter. It takes effort to create and nurture good connections. Make them a priority.
- Connect more with your food through how you shop, cook and eat.
- Finding or developing a spiritual connection (in whatever way that works for you) can be a key tool to optimise your health and happiness as you age.
- Deepening self-awareness and encouraging self-acceptance can increase resilience, happiness and fulfilment.
- Prioritise your needs, quieten your inner critics, set healthy boundaries, find more joy and gratitude, reframe your thoughts, and find your purpose

CHAPTER 12:

E – ELIMINATE and defend

The final 'E' in the EMBRACE protocol focuses on the health of our gut, liver and immune system. These organs are crucial not only for maintaining overall health but also for promoting healthy ageing.

The gut and liver are the unsung heroes of detoxification, working tirelessly to eliminate toxins and waste – an increasingly vital process as we age. Meanwhile, the immune system serves as the body's defence against illness, disease and accelerated ageing.

YOUR GUT

As we saw in Part 2, a healthy gut is foundational to our health and how we age. Going beyond simply digesting your food, your gut is a complex ecosystem, essentially acting as a 'second brain'. It's a control centre, regulating inflammation, your immune system, nutrient absorption, hormone production and even your mental health.

Your gut is a long tube that starts at your mouth and ends at your anus, working tirelessly to break down the food you eat, absorb essential nutrients and expel waste. Think of it as a bustling city with millions of inhabitants (your microbiome). These little helpers form a diverse community of microorganisms, including bacteria, viruses, fungi and other microbes, and they play a vital role in everything from digestion to immunity, and even influence your mood.

The National Institutes of Health state that within your gut microbiome, there are a whopping 8 million genes at play. To put it in perspective, this means your body hosts 360 times more bacterial genes than human genes!

Just as a well-run city relies on its community and services, a healthy body relies on a well-balanced gut with a strong lining. When this balance is off, it can trigger a chain reaction of health issues, from digestive troubles to hormone imbalances and immune dysfunction, affecting your overall wellbeing and crucially how well you age.

By midlife, your gut has taken a lot of abuse: from your diet (sugar, alcohol, processed or takeaway foods, low fibre, etc.), to stress, toxins, antibiotics and other medications. And then menopause, no surprise, has an impact. Your sex hormones aren't just about reproduction; they also interact with the gut microbiome, influencing how food is broken down, nutrients are absorbed, and even how fat is stored.

Equally there's a collection of microbes that influence how oestrogen is metabolised and used by the body (the 'oestrobolome'). Lower levels of sex hormones post menopause can upset this delicate balance, increasing the risk of varying digestive issues as well as weight gain and chronic diseases.

What's more, the gut-brain axis (the super communication highway) means that changes in gut health can have a knock-on effect on mental wellbeing. Your gut helps produce neurotransmitters like serotonin, which keeps your mood stable.

So, you see, it's all connected – your hormones, gut health, immune system and even your mental health are part of this intricate web, which becomes more crucial to manage during and beyond menopause.

What does a healthy microbiome do for us?

Nutrient absorption and digestion: Microbes assist in breaking down complex carbohydrates, fibre and proteins that our bodies can't digest on their own – and they help in the absorption of essential nutrients.

Immune system: The microbiome interacts with immune cells, helping them to identify harmful pathogens. This interaction is crucial for developing and maintaining a robust immune response.

Synthesis of vitamins: Gut bacteria synthesise certain vitamins, notably vitamin K and some B vitamins, which are essential for various bodily functions, including blood clotting and energy metabolism.

Gut barrier integrity: The microbiome helps maintain the integrity of the gut lining, acting as a barrier against harmful substances and pathogens. This is essential for preventing conditions like leaky gut syndrome, which can lead to inflammation, autoimmune conditions and other health issues.

Metabolic regulation: Gut bacteria influence metabolism and have been linked to the regulation of body weight and fat storage. Imbalances in the gut microbiome have been associated with metabolic disorders like obesity and type 2 diabetes.

Mental health and mood: Gut bacteria produce neurotransmitters and other chemicals that influence brain function and mood, potentially affecting conditions like depression and anxiety. It's thought as much as 90% of your serotonin is produced in the gut!

Inflammation reduction: A healthy gut microbiome can help regulate inflammation in the body, preventing chronic inflamm-aging.

Microbiome diversity seems to be a key differential. Recent research found that older adults with a more unique pattern of changes in their gut microbiome were found to be healthier and have longer lifespans compared to those with less microbiome diversity

Bacteria can process information and communicate rapidly, even impacting your thoughts and actions. That's why it's important to give your gut bugs the right kind of food.

As well as the general gut health tips I covered in Part 2 (Happy gut, happy you), here are some tips to look after your microbiome.

Mix it up: Increasing the variety of foods in your diet is a great way to improve the diversity of your gut microbiome. Include a wide range of fruits, vegetables, legumes, nuts, seeds and whole grains in your diet. Each type of plant and each colour contain different phytonutrients that beneficial gut bacteria thrive on. Try to incorporate a variety of colours and different herbs and spices in your meals. Consider a weekly organic veg delivery box to liven up your usual shop and encourage you to cook with new (and seasonal) ingredients.

Add more fibre: Fibre is an all-round superhero for your microbiome! It acts as a prebiotic, feeding the good bacteria, which ferment the fibre, producing short-chain fatty acids (SCFAs) like butyrate, which is vital for gut barrier function and has anti-inflammatory properties, which are particularly beneficial as the body's immune response changes post menopause. Fibre also helps with regular bowel movements and preventing constipation, and it contributes to a more diverse and resilient gut microbiome. And it's been shown to help you live longer. A study published in the American Journal of Epidemiology in 2015 showed that for every additional 10g of fibre consumed per day, the risk of dying decreased by 10%.

Aim for a minimum of 35g a day. Here's the average fibre content of some common foods:

1 apple (5g)
1 banana (3g)
1 avocado (9g)
1 cup lentils (15g)
½ cup almonds (6g)
2 tbsp flaxseeds (5g) or 1 tbsp chia seeds (5g)
1 cup broccoli or carrots (5g)
1 cup blueberries (4g) or 1 cup raspberries (8g)
1 cup black beans (16g)
1 cup quinoa (5g)
1 cup cooked oatmeal (4g)
1 cup chickpeas (28g)
1 cup peanuts or peanut butter (14g)

Prebiotics: These are foods that feed your good gut bacteria, particularly species like Bifidobacteria and Lactobacilli. By feeding these helpful microbes, prebiotics help them thrive and multiply, leading to a more balanced and diverse gut flora. Prebiotic-rich foods include garlic, onions, leeks and asparagus. Green bananas and cold cooked potatoes, which contain 'resistant starch', are also favourite foods for your bugs. Prebiotic supplements often contain key components like inulin, fructo-oligosaccharides (FOS), galacto-oligosaccharides (GOS), resistant starch, xylo-oligosaccharides (XOS), polydextrose and arabinogalactans, all of which are known to nourish and promote the growth of beneficial gut bacteria.

Probiotics: These friendly bacteria play a key role in maintaining a healthy gut microbiome, ensuring everything from effective digestion to robust immune function. By populating the gut with good bacteria, probiotics help fend off harmful microbes and reinforce the intestinal barrier, acting as a first line of defence against inflammation and infections. Probiotic-rich foods include natural yoghurt, kefir, sauerkraut, kimchi, kombucha, miso and homemade sourdough bread. Supplements can be helpful but unless you can see a health practitioner for personalised advice (there are millions of different strains), you're better off getting your probiotics through food.

If you have to take a course of antibiotics, make sure you balance it with some good-quality probiotics. It won't affect your antibiotics if you take them separately (e.g. antibiotic in the morning, probiotic at night).

Remember, changes don't have to be made overnight – even small, incremental additions to support your gut can make a significant difference.

Oral health

Oral health isn't just about nice teeth and avoiding bad breath; your mouth is the gateway to your gastrointestinal tract, and like it or not, is home to a whole community of microorganisms including bacteria, fungi and viruses. This complex ecosystem is known as the oral microbiota and just like the gut microbiota, a healthy balance of bacteria in your mouth is essential to protect against infection, aid digestion and support your immune system.

If there's any imbalance, harmful bacteria can spread throughout the body and contribute to various health conditions, including cardiovascular disease, diabetes and respiratory infections. Several studies have shown an association between gum disease and increased risk of certain cancers. And there's growing evidence that it could also be linked with Alzheimer's disease.

So, we need to practise good oral hygiene every day. This includes regular brushing (electric brushes remove more plaque than manual ones) and flossing to remove plaque and food particles (I use a water flosser), as well as routine dental check-ups for professional cleanings and early detection of any oral health issues.

Additionally, adopting a balanced diet, limiting sugary and acidic foods and drinks, and avoiding smoking can further support oral health and bacterial balance.

Be careful with the regular use of commercial mouthwashes – they can be useful for specific dental issues, but they can disrupt the beneficial bacteria that are essential for maintaining oral and overall health. And make sure your toothpaste doesn't include potentially harmful ingredients such as triclosan, SLS, artificial sweeteners, dyes and microbeads.

YOUR LIVER

It's an amazing thing, your liver. Did you know it's the largest organ in the body, weighing over four pounds? And that it has over 500 jobs to do?

Your liver is under more strain than ever before. In recent decades, it has had to contend with thousands of new chemicals found in the air we breathe, the food we eat, the products we use, and the water we drink – not to mention that nightly glass or two of wine!

When your liver struggles to keep up, toxins and waste can accumulate, much like a vacuum bag full of dust, and may be recirculated into your bloodstream. Poor liver health can result in impaired nutrient metabolism, hormone imbalances and an increased risk of chronic diseases such as liver cirrhosis, fatty liver disease, and diabetes – all of which can accelerate ageing and deteriorate overall health.

The chemical soup we live in

In the last 100 years or so, the amount of chemicals used in modern manufacture has skyrocketed. Growing evidence is showing that our exposure to many of these chemicals has contributed to chronic disease and hormonal conditions.

Our bodies are designed to handle a certain amount of toxins, but they are increasingly struggling to cope with the cumulative effect of all these new chemicals. Our genes play a huge part in how well we detoxify, and some people can tolerate numerous toxins with no apparent effects. However, for many of us, these chemicals can cause disruption and pose a risk to our health as we age.

In 2024, researchers tracked 257 patients over 34 months, finding that 150 of them had polyethylene in their blood. These patients showed higher levels of inflammation and less collagen in their blood vessels, indicating potential damage to their vascular structure. Surprisingly, those with microplastics in their plaques were 4.53 times more likely to experience severe cardiovascular events or death.

We've known for decades about a group of chemicals called endocrine-disrupting chemicals or EDCs. They are molecularly similar to certain hormones, making it difficult for our bodies to distinguish between the real and the fake. These chemicals can play tricks on us by increasing certain hormones, decreasing others, mimicking hormones, transforming one hormone into another, interfering with hormone signalling, competing with essential nutrients, binding to hormones, and accumulating in organs that produce hormones – all of which can contribute to many more serious issues. According to the World Health Organization, the vast majority of chemicals that interfere with our hormones have not even been tested.

In 2009, the USA Endocrine Society issued a scientific statement expressing concern about endocrine-disrupting chemicals (EDCs) and the serious health problems they can cause, including cancer, heart disease, diabetes, PCOS, obesity, thyroid disease, and reproductive issues.

Toxins don't just disrupt our hormones, they can damage our cells and DNA in every part of our bodies, potentially causing health issues and accelerating ageing.

Where are these chemicals lurking?

Everywhere! But when you can't see them, it's not easy to know about them. They're in:

- the air we breathe
- the food we eat, and the water we drink (e.g. pesticides, heavy metals, plastic)
- our household products that we use in the home (e.g. air fresheners, scented candles, cleaning and laundry products, fire retardants, kitchenware)
- our beauty and personal products that we inhale or put on our skin (e.g. perfume, body lotion, cosmetics, shampoo, shower gel, sunscreen, deodorant, etc.)

What are the big ones to avoid?

BPA and microplastics: You probably know about BPA. It's one of the most researched endocrine disrupting chemicals. It's in everything plastic, from water bottles to food containers, to till receipts and tin can linings. Research found it in the blood of 96% of pregnant women! BPA has been linked to everything from breast to reproductive problems, obesity, early puberty and heart disease.

Microplastics on the other hand are fairly new to scientific health research. They are tiny plastic particles ranging in size from less than five millimetres (microplastics) to less than one-thousandth of a millimetre (nanoplastics). We primarily ingest them through contaminated food (especially seafood) and drinks in plastic bottles, but also through the air and skin. Recently, microplastics and nanoplastics have been found in human brains, hearts, lungs and arteries, potentially contributing to cardiovascular disease. They have also been detected in breast milk, the placenta and even penises! We don't yet know the full extent of the impact of this, but so far studies are showing links to inflammation, oxidative stress, cellular damage and cardiovascular disease.

Swap to glass or stainless steel where you can. Minimise use of plastic water bottles, food containers, plastic wrap, tins and cans (especially acidic foods like tomatoes, soups, sodas, ready meals). BPA can leach into food and drink particularly when heated, so avoid putting any plastic into the microwave or oven.

PVC (polyvinyl chloride colon PVC): PVC releases toxic chemicals like dioxins and phthalates, which can lead to serious health issues including respiratory problems, hormonal disruptions, and increased cancer risk. Commonly found in pipes and plumbing fixtures, vinyl flooring and various consumer goods like vinyl shower curtains, toys and packaging materials (e.g. clingfilm).

Switch to non-PVC clingfilm, wax food coverings and cotton shower curtains.

Pesticides: When something is invented to kill living insects, you know it can't be good for the living microbes inside of us either. Despite many studies linking organophosphate pesticide exposure to numerous health issues, they are still among the more common pesticides in use today. They are linked to thyroid cancer, ADHD, leukaemia, birth defects, fertility problems and a host more health issues.

Eat organic where possible, especially when you're eating the skins of products (e.g. salad leaves, fruit).

Phthalates: A group of chemicals found in synthetic fragrance and plastic products, studies have linked phthalates to hormone conditions, infertility, birth defects, obesity, diabetes and thyroid issues. Fragrance is particularly pervasive in our lives. We're talking about any products that smell nice, from perfume, to scented candles, air fresheners, cleaning and laundry products, skincare, hair products and more. Inhaling phthalates is the quickest way into the bloodstream, so look for products made from essential oils instead.

Check for 'fragrance' or 'parfum' listed in the ingredients of many products (this means it's synthetic). If it has a strong smell and it's not made from essential oils, it's likely to be there.
If you can't live without your favourite perfume, spray it on your clothes instead of your skin (and do it with the window open).

There are some amazing natural brands out there now including some of my favourites: Tropic, Get Fussy natural deodorants, By Sarah, Neals Yard, Green People, Weleda, Dr Bronner's, Burt's Bees, Dr Hauschka – and many more.

Perfluorinated chemicals (PFCs): Often referred to as 'forever chemicals' because they are very hard to degrade and can stay in the body for a long time. They are mostly found in non-stick cookware (e.g. Teflon), food packaging, stain and water repellents (e.g. Scotchguard and Gore-Tex). Associated health issues include decreased sperm quality, low birth weight, kidney disease, thyroid disease and high cholesterol.

Replace your non-stick cookware with ceramic or stainless steel (use more olive oil or coconut oil to prevent sticking!).

Triclosan: Found in antibacterial handwashes and popular toothpaste brands, triclosan has been shown to interfere with thyroid function, which could lead to neurological and behavioural problems.

Ditch all antibacterial personal care products – numerous studies have shown that soap and water is just as effective. Check the active ingredients in your toothpaste and switch if necessary.

PBBs (polybrominated biphenols): Found in chemical flame retardants used on sofas, mattresses, carpets, cars, furniture, clothing, and associated with cancers, birth defects and developmental effects in developing foetuses. The UK government has recently proposed new regulations to enable safer methods to meet fire safety regulations.

VOCs (volatile organic compounds): Such as benzene, formaldehyde, toluene or perchloroethylene. They are found in dry cleaning chemicals, solvents, glue, nail varnish, cleaning sprays (check for limonene). When they evaporate, we inhale them. VOCs have been linked with cancer, liver and kidney disease, among other serious health conditions.

Limit your dry cleaning and air your clothes fully afterwards, switch to natural nail care brands and cleaning products.

Heavy metals: lead, mercury, arsenic: As well as a host of general health issues, these heavy metals are also linked to hormone disruption. Lead (found in some paint, lipstick and tap water), arsenic (tap water, some rice products), aluminium (in many antiperspirants/deodorants) and mercury (amalgam fillings, water, large fish) are best avoided where possible.

UV filters (commonly found in sunscreen): In 2021, the FDA in the US declared that 12 ingredients commonly found in sunscreen products were not generally recognised as safe and effective due to insufficient data: avobenzone, cinoxate, dioxybenzone, ensulizole, homosalate, meradimate, octinoxate, octisalate, octocrylene, oxybenzone, padimate O and sulisobenzone. Mineral sunscreens that contain titanium dioxide and zinc oxide are generally considered a much safer option, although it's best to avoid powders and sprays as inhaling nanoparticles can also be harmful.

If you can, do a thorough review of your environment and the products around you. We can't avoid these chemicals completely, but we can do an awful lot to minimise our exposure, and supporting your liver will help to detoxify the ones you can't avoid.

I'm not asking you to change everything, that would be overwhelming! Just be aware of the chemicals you may be inhaling, eating, drinking or putting on your skin.

Don't just take my word for it, do some research and check it out for yourself. I know how hard it is to give up products you have been using for years. But just making a start is enough, and you can do it slowly. Just change one product at a time. It won't be long before you're seriously minimising your exposure and giving your body a nice detox!

So, what else can we do to best look after our liver?

- **Hydrate, hydrate, hydrate!** Staying hydrated helps your liver work properly. Head back to Eat for more tips on keeping topped up.
- **Drink less alcohol.** Whether you are ditching alcohol for good, or just reducing your intake, it's going to help your liver.
- **Eat more broccoli ...** and cauliflower, kale, cabbage, Brussels sprouts, rocket, watercress. They are all cruciferous veg that can help your liver to detoxify more efficiently.
- **Ditch the sugar, refined carbs and processed foods.** Stressing out your liver with too much sugar (that includes refined carbs) and industrial fats is going to raise insulin, cortisol and oestrogen – not good news for your liver.
- **Eat enough protein.** Protein helps your liver do its job. Revisit the Eat section for all the info on protein.
- **Eat more nuts.** Nuts help to reduce oxidative stress, especially walnuts. A few Brazil nuts a day will also help provide selenium and glutathione – powerful antioxidants!
- **Get your bowels moving.** If you're constipated, toxic waste can build up in your gut, so eat plenty of fibre, supplement with magnesium (citrate is best for relaxing the bowel), drink plenty of water and exercise daily.
- **Watch the pill popping.** Don't just pop a pill without thought. Your liver has to detox any kind of medication, including antibiotics, paracetamol, ibuprofen, birth control pills and indigestion tablets.
- **Get a good nights' sleep.** While we are sleeping, the liver is hard at work detoxifying our day. What's more, even a single nights' bad sleep can impact our liver function. Jump back to my sleep tips in Part 2 and Rest for more help.
- **Get sweating!** Your skin is one of your most important detoxification organs, so sweating is a good way to get rid of toxins. Exercise, saunas, steam rooms, hot baths – try anything that gets you sweating (and ticking the self-care/ move box too).
- **Supplement.** Take a good daily multi for your basics, and add in some magnesium, glutathione or NAC, or a good liver formula to support you.

YOUR IMMUNE SYSTEM

Your immune system is not just important for preventing colds and infections, it's your whole defence against disease and ageing – your army, navy and airforce fighting anything that might damage you, externally and internally.

It helps keep you safe from environmental pathogens (viruses, bacteria), toxins, pollution. It also fights off any nasties that you might eat or drink, making sure they are eliminated safely. And it repairs you if you injure yourself, rushing specialised repair cells to the scene of damage, fixing it up and minimising any further danger.

The immune system plays a vital role in protecting against chronic diseases like heart disease, cancer and dementia through various mechanisms. It regulates inflammation, which is pivotal in preventing chronic disease. It uses specialised cells, such as natural killer cells and cytotoxic T cells, to detect and eliminate cancerous cells, preventing the formation of tumours. It aids in DNA repair, attacks harmful free radicals and reduces oxidative stress. Additionally, the brain's immune surveillance system, involving microglia, helps clear waste products that can cause neurodegenerative conditions.

A well-regulated immune response also prevents autoimmune diseases and maintains cardiovascular health by reducing inflammation and repairing vessel damage.

Interestingly, some of the key pathways of ageing, such as cellular senescence, chronic inflammation and compromised autophagy (the body's cellular 'clean-up' process), are closely intertwined with how our immune system functions. And as we get older, our immune system ages and we can become less resilient and more susceptible to illness, infection, disease, autoimmune conditions and accelerated ageing. Scientists call this progressive deterioration in immune function, 'immunosenescence'.

Despite the advances of modern science and medicine, nutrition and lifestyle interventions are still one of the most powerful ways to ensure the resilience of your immune system.

We looked at how to strengthen your immune system in Part 2 through your diet, stress management, sleep, exercise and targeted supplements.

What are some more targeted strategies?

Diet: Specific foods for immune function include:
- Mushrooms (reishi, shitake) – beta glucans within these mushroom types have been shown to support white blood cell function.
- Garlic, onions, ginger – all have antimicrobial properties.
- Spices (turmeric, rosemary, oregano) – these are anti-inflammatory.
- Fermented foods (e.g. sauerkraut, live yoghurt, kefir, kombucha) – these include probiotics for gut support.
- Hydration – important to keep your immune cells hydrated. You can include coffee in moderation for the antioxidant content.

Cold exposure: In the Activate section, we discussed the health benefits of regular cold exposure. Incorporating this practice consistently can be particularly advantageous for enhancing our immune system.

When we expose ourselves to cold temperatures (for example, a cold shower, ice bath or wild swim), our body initiates a cold shock response, triggering various physiological changes. This controlled exposure to cold harnesses something called 'hormesis', where small doses of stressors like cold enhance our health and resilience. It involves the release of norepinephrine, a stress hormone, which inhibits inflammatory cytokines and activates the fight-or-flight response.

On a microscopic level, cold therapy boosts immune cells like natural killer cells and cytotoxic T cells, while also enhancing antioxidant defences and regulating proteins associated with inflammation. Additionally, it promotes lymphatic drainage, improving the efficiency of waste removal and enhancing white blood cell activity. The real-world benefits include reduced infection, improved resilience and even conscious control over immune responses.

You might be acquainted with the groundbreaking study featuring Wim Hof, who was injected with a strain of E. coli but consciously regulated his immune system to reject the infection through meditation, deep breathing and cold-water therapy. Some thought it was some kind of fluke, but the results have been reproduced in a Dutch study.

Cold water therapy isn't just for the brave souls taking hour-long ice baths. Even small doses of cold exposure can yield impressive results, from reducing common illnesses to alleviating more serious conditions and granting us conscious control over our immune system responses.

Meditation: We have known for a while that meditation can play a significant role in enhancing various aspects of immune function, however a study in 2023 showed how meditation can elevate SERPINA5, a gene that helps block viruses entering our cells (in this case it was Covid-19). And we know from Dr Joe Dispenza's research about the incredible power of the mind to heal our bodies.

SUMMARY

- A well-functioning gut microbiome and a healthy liver are key to reducing the risk of chronic disease as we age.
- Feed your microbiome with diverse plants, prebiotic and probiotic foods with plenty of fibre.
- Look after your oral health through proper brushing and flossing, and regular check-ups.
- Your liver health is under attack. Look after it by minimising environmental chemicals and toxins, and supporting it through your diet and lifestyle choices.
- A properly functioning immune system is equally crucial in protecting the body by regulating inflammation, detecting and eliminating cancerous cells, repairing DNA and maintaining overall tissue and organ health.
- Support your immune system through diet and lifestyle interventions, adding in cold exposure and meditation to enhance resilience.

CHAPTER 13:

BEYOND EMBRACE

Now that you have the tools for living a healthy and happy life after menopause, in this section I'll show you how you can delve a bit deeper and optimise your health through a more personalised approach using health testing and 1-1 support.

TESTING AND SUPPORT

I have alluded to health testing in various parts of this book. If you're suffering from health issues or symptoms and you still don't have answers, getting the right tests done can often be the missing link.

Every BODY is unique. This is why the one-size-fits-all standard medical approach doesn't work for everyone. Working with a qualified nutritionist or practitioner can help you get to the root cause of the issue, rather than just manage your symptoms.

Getting regular tests carried out can amplify your healthy ageing strategy. Here's a selection of tests that have proved vital in our work with women over the past ten years:

Hormones
I've talked about your Feisty Four hormones and how important they are in how you feel. Getting these tested can be really helpful to identifying where any imbalances may lie:

Cortisol:
The standard medical approach typically relies on single blood samples and is very much limited to diagnosing specific

medical conditions like Cushing's syndrome or Addison's disease.

Private testing often utilises urine or saliva samples and offers a more comprehensive view of cortisol levels over time, allowing for frequent monitoring. This approach enables individuals to assess cortisol fluctuations throughout the day or across several days, making it valuable for stress management, hormonal balance evaluation and overall health optimisation, providing a more detailed picture of cortisol patterns and potential imbalances.

Insulin:
Standard medical testing for insulin typically involves obtaining a blood sample, providing a single-point measurement of insulin levels primarily for diagnosing diabetes or evaluating specific medical conditions. A standard HbA1c test at your doctor (or privately) will measure your 'glycated' haemoglobin, a measure of how much 'sticky blood' you have. This is seen as a marker for pre-diabetes or diabetes.

Thyroid:
As I mentioned in the Balance section, standard medical tests for thyroid function typically involve blood tests, which assess specific thyroid hormone levels, such as TSH (thyroid-stimulating hormone) and T4 (thyroxine). These tests do not always include T3, the active thyroid hormone, or thyroid antibodies. And reference ranges are very wide, so borderline or low levels may not qualify for treatment but may still cause symptoms.

Private thyroid testing not only measures active thyroid hormone levels but also evaluates thyroid antibodies, reverse T3, and other thyroid-related markers. These panels provide a more thorough assessment of thyroid function and potential autoimmune thyroid conditions which can provide a much more targeted treatment protocol. Private testing is particularly helpful for those who are on medication but still having symptoms, or if you've been told your results are 'normal' or 'borderline'.

Sex Hormones:
Standard medical testing typically involves blood tests to measure specific hormones like oestradiol (a form of oestrogen), progesterone and testosterone. These tests are not routine, even when prescribing medication such as HRT, as they may not always provide a comprehensive overview of sex hormone levels or consider individual variations.

Private sex hormone testing often includes comprehensive hormone panels using urine samples that measure a broader range of hormones, including different forms of oestrogen (e.g. oestriol and oestrone), free and total testosterone, progesterone, DHEA and their metabolites. These panels offer a more in-depth assessment of sex hormone status and behaviour over a 24-hour period, making them valuable for individuals interested in optimising hormonal balance, or addressing specific hormonal concerns.

Gut health

If you suffer from digestive issues or IBS, it can be really hard to get to the root cause. Standard medical tests typically involve stool tests that assess for specific markers like faecal occult blood, pathogens or parasites. These tests are typically conducted when there are clinical symptoms or concerns related to gastrointestinal issues. They focus on identifying and addressing acute problems or infections.

Private gut health testing, such as comprehensive microbiome analysis, goes beyond the standard tests by examining the diversity and composition of the gut microbiota as well as inflammation markers and enzyme status. These tests provide a detailed profile of the microbiome and potential impact on overall health. It's a much more holistic view of gut health, allowing you to gain insights into the balance of beneficial and harmful bacteria, digestive function, and explore potential connections between gut health and your symptoms. It is especially valuable for those interested in proactive measures to optimise their digestive health and overall wellness.

Brain health

If you suffer from brain fog, memory issues or are worried about dementia or Alzheimer's disease as you get older, you may want to consider some key tests to measure brain health. These include vitamin D, vitamin B12, omega-3 fats, HbA1c, homocysteine and glutathione.

Standard medical blood tests might look at some of these, such as HbA1c, vitamin D, vitamin B12 and iron, but private testing can offer specialised tests such as omega-3 fats, homocysteine and glutathione. Results can then determine where you may want to focus your diet and supplement needs.

Inflammation

It's difficult to test for inflammation in any one area, but there are general blood markers you want to look out for, including:

- **C-reactive protein (or CRP):** This test can tell you if there's an excess of inflammation in your body, but it can't pinpoint the exact source.
- **Ferritin:** High levels of iron stores can indicate inflammation.
- **HbA1c:** High levels are a risk factor for insulin resistance and type 2 diabetes, both indicators of high inflammation.
- **Vitamin D:** Low levels increase the risk of inflammation.
- **Thyroid (TSH, T4, T3 and antibodies):** Low thyroid hormones and high antibodies can identify an autoimmune condition.

Heart Health

If you've been told you have high cholesterol, consider checking some of these markers to get a more comprehensive picture of your heart health:

- **Thyroid panel:** TSH, T4, T3 and antibodies.
- **CRP (C-Reactive Protein):** A marker for inflammation.
- **Fibrinogen:** Elevated levels can indicate increased clotting and higher risk of CVD.
- **Homocysteine:** High levels are associated with arterial

damage and a higher risk of heart diseases.

- **LDL particle size and number:** Not all LDL particles pose the same risk. Small, dense LDL particles are more atherogenic than larger, buoyant LDL particles.
- **Triglycerides (TGs):** High triglyceride levels are associated with increased CVD risk, particularly when HDL is low.
- **Glycated hemoglobin (HbA1c):** Elevated levels may indicate poor glucose control, increasing the risk of heart disease in diabetics and possibly in non-diabetics as well.
- **Insulin resistance markers:** Tests like fasting insulin levels and HOMA-IR can assess your insulin sensitivity, which can be a precursor to type 2 diabetes and is associated with higher cardiovascular risk.
- **Sex hormones:** Oestrogen, progesterone, testosterone.
- **Blood pressure:** Hypertension is a significant risk factor for heart disease and stroke.
- **BMI and waist circumference:** While not blood markers, these measurements can indicate obesity, a risk factor for CVD.
- **Infection:** For example, H. pylori, herpes and SIBO can result in higher LDL levels.
- **Genetic tests:** Some people are genetically predisposed to higher cholesterol or CVD risk. Specific gene tests can sometimes add valuable context.

Some of these you will be able to request via your doctor, however others are only available privately.

Nutrients
Health testing for key nutrients such as vitamin D, vitamin B12, iron, magnesium, omega-3 fats and others can be really helpful to identify deficiencies or imbalances, allowing for personalised dietary adjustments and supplementation to support overall wellbeing and prevent potential health issues.

If you're not able to get these done via standard medical testing, you can get home testing kits that are easy to do.

DNA

DNA testing, also known as genetic testing or nutrigenomic testing, offers a personalised approach to understanding your genetic predispositions and potential health risks. These tests offer a unique insight into your genetic profile allowing practitioners to create a gene-based healthy eating plan, dietary goals for relevant vitamins, minerals, phytochemicals, and foods and supplement recommendations.

DNA testing can provide unique insights into various health areas, such as fat and carbohydrate metabolism, helping to identify your ideal diet. It can assess heart disease risk by examining the impact of cholesterol on cardiovascular health and evaluate B vitamins (B6, B12 and folate) involved in DNA and cell renewal. It can identify processes related to calcium and vitamin D metabolism for bone health, analyse phase 1 and phase 2 enzyme functions for detoxification, and determine your body's inflammatory response to injury, infection and allergies. It also offers insights into insulin resistance by examining cell insulin sensitivity, aiding in the management of metabolic health.

If you have any symptoms or health issues that haven't been identified or that you'd like to go deeper on to find the root cause, then it would be worth considering getting some testing done. If you are not able to access this through standard medical testing, there are many private practitioners and doctors that offer this, and you are welcome to contact us at www.happyhormonesforlife.com/contact for more information.

FINAL WORDS

Phew! If you're still with me, well done! We've gone through a lot here in this book. I really hope you're feeling inspired to take some action towards your own healthy ageing plan.

I've given you some tools to help you feel your best so you can make the most of your next phase. Now it's up to you to start taking action, stay vigilant, be your own advocate, listen to your body and have control over your health.

I said at the start of this book that this is your time, your chance to shine. But it's also your responsibility. Nobody knows your body better than you do. Take advice and medical help where you need to, but don't leave what's ultimately right for you and your body up to anyone else.

Some doctors do give diet and lifestyle advice, but training at medical school in nutrition, lifestyle, menopause and the mind-body connection is hugely lacking – and all of these have huge impacts on our wellbeing. The culture of polypharmacy (taking a cocktail of different prescribed medications) is growing dangerously and healthcare systems around the world are often overburdened and under-resourced, and struggling to support our ageing populations.

Although many doctors and educators are doing great work to fill in the gaps, and the UK recently published guidelines for GPs about "Shared Decision Making" with patients, it's still up to us to educate ourselves and be as informed as possible about our own health. Then if we do need treatment we can work more collaboratively with our doctors and health practitioners.

If you're reading this and have no idea where to start, I recommend taking a step-by-step approach by exploring each section of the EMBRACE protocol. Download the Workbook (www.happyhormonesforlife.com/life) and start by selecting one actionable item from each section that resonates with you or feels attainable. By focusing on small, manageable changes, you can gradually incorporate healthier habits into your routine and make meaningful progress toward improving your overall wellbeing.

After choosing your seven actions, jot them down and sketch out a plan for how you'll tackle each one. Pick a start date and ask a family member or friend to help keep you accountable (even better, get them involved!).

This is in no way an exact science but as you start to figure out what your body and mind need, you'll get to know yourself better and develop a deeper understanding of which strategies are going to serve you best.

Make your health your no. 1 priority. Nothing matters more! If you give it the attention and importance it deserves, you'll find time and motivation to create good habits. If not, you'll find excuses.

However, I don't want to encourage obsession around this. I've seen how easy it is for that to happen. Social media and health gurus have made 'biohacking' a real trend for those interested in longevity. And it feeds into our need for control, and our fear of ageing and mortality.

There's nothing wrong with experimenting and trying new things (I am encouraging that), but if any of it causes you to be miserable, to miss out on vital social connections, or cause you anxiety, then it's definitely not worth it. Balance is everything, otherwise we risk causing the health issues that we're trying to avoid!

We want to be doing what we can to feel good, but not at any cost. Feeling relaxed and happy is more important than obsessing about living forever. Knowledge can be powerful, but it can also cause unnecessary worry. There are some things we just can't control.

And remember, no woman's journey is the same. There is no magic way to live your life, whatever anyone tells you. You must find your unique blueprint and complete your own jigsaw puzzle of health and wellbeing. But stay flexible. What works for you in your 50s may not work in your 60s or beyond. Stay vigilant and adapt your protocols whenever you need.

Mine is complete – for now. But I know I need to keep reviewing it. My body is constantly transforming, as is science and knowledge, especially in the field of ageing. And life happens. So, I need to be adaptable and willing to be open to new ideas and changes to my plan.

I recommend you stay open too. And be ready to discover new joy in these bonus years that we are privileged to experience. If we prioritise taking care of our physical and emotional health now, we'll keep our bodies healthy and thriving as we age. With that and a bit of luck, we'll age better, feel less pain and stay out of the healthcare system for as long as possible.

Finally, let's recognise and appreciate what numerous cultures have long understood: menopause can be a deeply meaningful and spiritual phase in our lives, symbolising a transition from the old self to the most empowered versions of ourselves we have ever been.

Thank you for coming on this journey with me, and I will leave you with some inspirational words that I've picked up while writing this book.

WORDS TO INSPIRE

66Whenever you feel afraid, just remember. Courage is the root of change – and change is what we're chemically designed to do. So when you wake up tomorrow, make this pledge. No more holding yourself back. No more subscribing to others' opinions of what you can and cannot achieve. And no more allowing anyone to pigeonhole you into useless categories of sex, race, economic status and religion. Do not allow your talents to lie dormant, ladies. Design your own future. When you go home today, ask yourself what YOU will change. And then get started.99
Excerpt from Lessons in Chemistry by Bonnie Garmus (another inspirational woman, who published this, her first book, at age 62).

66So perhaps it's time to throw away the doubts on what we think we can and can't do, what we should and shouldn't achieve, and who we may or may not be, and open the windows of our soul to the sun. To stop holding ourselves back and to allow the change, whether that be a tumultuous plate shift or a gentle nudge in a new direction, to let go, and to do it with extraordinary love.
The only way we can fail is by giving up.99
Emma Simpson, www.emmasimpsonauthor.com

66Mid-life is a time where the old is burned off, and even though our waistlines grow, the bare bones of us are exposed.
The raw, naked guts of us, if we're willing.
I'm willing.
I'm tired of the bullshit, the people-pleasing, the tolerating, the constant fucking tolerating.
Being 'nice', making sure they like me, making sure no one gets upset, hoping they don't all leave me.
I used to think of it as a gentle unfolding of our hearts, but

today it feels much more visceral than that, a ripping open of the chest and exposing the rawness, the absolute vulnerability of me.

There's sheer power there, inside, bottled up for all these years. Dangerous power if unharnessed but just for a moment, letting it out to career around – the image of a woman, stripped naked, in the moonlight, head thrown back and arms thrown wide saying 'yes'.

And as all the coverings are burned away, what is left is beauty and purpose.

Finally free to do what I came here to do.

Not, actually, much to my surprise, to be here in service.

But be here to be myself.

And only that.

Because it is everything.

I'll lose friends and fans; I'm sure.

I never felt truly myself around them anyway.

I've have never truly felt like myself for the past forty-five years.

I didn't fit in, I wasn't enough, I tried so hard, I wanted desperately to be noticed, I was always on the outside – only now I'm claiming all of it.

Yes, I cry. Yes, I feel lonely. Yes, I feel angry. Yes, I feel deep, bitter sadness. Yes, I especially feel rage.

And don't dare try to offer sympathy, make me feel better or even extend me kindness.

This part I have to do alone.

Be in the fire. Be with the fire. BE the fire.

Until all of the excess is gone and I can discover what is left.

Fuck, I'm so grateful to be a woman. That I get to make this transition and start anew.

I thought I would make my way through this change with grace; kind of spiritually and in a zen, floaty self-righteous manner, slowly greying and becoming peaceful.

I did not expect the street-fighting, the dirt and the blood and the ugliness of it all.

And yet here it is, out on the page for all to see.

There.

It's done now.

This crazy mad woman outed.
Burn too, fellow mad-women.
Let's find out who you really are.**"**

Nicola Bird, www.nicolabird.net

"It's never too late.
In an instant you can make a new decision.
That's the micro-leap moment.
In that instant, you can take your life in a new direction.
Your life doesn't happen in the past or the future.
Your life happens in the present.
Right here.
Right now.
Now is where you make a decision and take action.
Now is where you decide it's not too late to begin a life.**"**

Suzy Walker, www.suzywalker.com

RESOURCES

HAPPY HORMONES FOR LIFE
Website; www.happyhormonesforlife.com
For free resources, self-help options or information on the
health tests and 1-1 support available.

Social media:
IG @happyhormonesforlife
FB: @happyhormonesforlife
LI: @williamsnicki

Recommended brands:
www.happyhormonesforlife.com/recommendations – for some
of our favourite brands and products.
Book resources:
www.happyhormonesforlife.com/life – including the Life After
Menopause workbook and references.

Mental health and trauma:
Victim Support: www.victimsupport.org.uk
Mind: www.mind.org.uk
Samaritans: a helpline available 24/7 – 116 123
Women's Aid: helpline – 0808 2000 247

Loneliness:
Campaign to End Loneliness: www.campaigntoendloneliness.org
Age UK: www.ageuk.org.uk
The Silver Line: a free helpline available 24/7 for older adults in
the UK – 0800 4 70 80 90
British Association for Counselling and Psychotherapy (BACP):
www.bacp.co.uk

Families, children and relationships:
Fertility Network UK: www.fertilitynetworkuk.org
Home-Start UK: www.home-start.org.uk
Family Lives: www.familylives.org.uk

Grief/bereavement:
Cruse Bereavement Care: www.cruse.org.uk
The Compassionate Friends: www.tcf.org.uk

Volunteering:
National Council for Voluntary organisations: www.ncvo.org.uk
Volunteer Match: www.volunteermatch.com

Health websites:
Institute of Functional Medicine: www.ifm.org
Brain health: www.foodforthebrain.org
Sleep: www.drnerina.com
HeartMath: www.heartmath.com
Balance Menopause App (Dr Louise Newson): www.balance-menopause.com/dr-louise-newson
Liminal; supplements and community: www.liveliminal.com
Environmental Working Group: www.ewg.org
Pesticide Action Network: www.pan-uk.org
Latte Lounge: www.lattelounge.co.uk
Katharine Gale, Menopause Clinic: www.fluxstate.co.uk
Hypnotherapy (especially for pain and anxiety): www.nickyelmer.co.uk
Disordered or emotional eating: www.marcellerosenutrition.co.uk
Herbalists: www.rachelboon.co.uk and www.melindamcdougall.com
Digital wellbeing: www.laura-willis.com

Self development:
HeartLeap with Suzy Walker: www.heartleap.substack.com
Something More with Caroline Ferguson: www.carolineferguson.substack.com
Dr Joe Dispenza: www.drjoedispenza.com
Brene Brown: www.brenebrown.com
Dr Joanna Martin and One of Many: www.oneofmany.co.uk
Tamu Thomas; www.livethreesixty.com
Menopause Whilst Black Podcast: www.thekarenarthur.com

Helpful books

The Upgrade, Dr Louann Brizendine
Breathe, James Nastor
Breaking the Habit of Being Yourself, Dr Joe Dispenza
Supernatural, by Dr Joe Dispenza
The Biology of Belief, Bruce Lipton
When the Body Says No: Understanding the Stress-Disease Connection, Gabor Mate
Age Proof, Professor Rose Anne Kenny
This Chair Rocks, Ashton Applewhite
Hagitude, Sharon Blackie
Forever Young, Dr Mark Hyman
You Can Be Younger, Marisa Peer
Ageless Body, Timeless Mind, Deepak Chopra
The Blue Zones, Dan Buettner
Atomic Habits, James Clear
The Power Decade, Susan Saunders
Upgrade Your Brain, Patrick Holford
The Stress Solution, Dr Rangan Chatterjee
Playing Big, Tara Mohr
The Telomere Effect, Dr Elizabeth Blackburn and Dr Elissa Epel
The Burnout Bible, Rachel Philpotts
Rushing Woman's Syndrome, Dr Libby Weaver
Unstressable, Mo Gawdat
Metabolical: The lure and the lies of processed food, nutrition and modern medicine, Robert Lustig
Sweet Poison, David Gillespie
The Glucose Goddess Method, Jesse Inchauspe
Ultra Processed People: Why do we eat stuff that isn't food … and why can't we stop?, Chris van Tulleken
The Artist's Way, Julia Cameron
Women Who Work Too Much, Tamu Thomas
Superwoman; Escaping the Myth, Dr Joanna Martin

ACKNOWLEDGEMENTS

A book like this doesn't get written without help and a support network.

It's a cliché but my husband Nigel is my absolute rock. He saw this book in me long before I knew I was capable of it. I realise how incredibly lucky we are to have found each other and share our lives together, along with his incredibly supportive family.

I'm also very fortunate that I am very close to my sister, brother and my 2 sisters-in-law, and both my parents. My dad, Dr Bernard Willis, was the one who set me off on this path, and I'm so very grateful to him. He's been a huge source of inspiration and support throughout my journey as a practitioner. At 80 years young, he is still seeing patients and is just as passionate today about helping people as he ever was.

I want to also thank my mum for being my biggest fan, and the source of several anecdotes throughout the book. At 79, her love of life, romance (she's on her 4th husband) and new adventures (she's on her 27th house) is never ending and a real inspiration to anyone who wants to live life to the full, at any age.

To my two kids, now adults: I am forever amazed and grateful for the incredible humans you have become. I can't express how proud I am.

To Lauren, Jo and all my Happy Hormones team, you have been a huge support to me in the last ten years – your hard work and commitment has allowed me the space and time to write the book. I thank you with all my heart.

To my wonderful friend Monica, and fellow NT's who have shared this journey with me, I couldn't have done this without your support.

And finally to the clients and community we have had the honour of supporting, you are the reason we do this work. I am always grateful for your trust in us, and your commitment to live a better life for yourself and others.

ABOUT THE AUTHOR

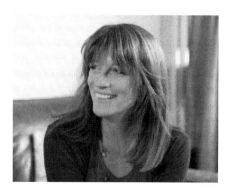

Nicki has been a leading voice and advocate of women's health for over a decade. After qualifying at the renowned Institute of Optimum Nutrition in 2014, Nicki founded Happy Hormones for Life to educate, inspire and empower women to reclaim their health and feel better than ever. In addition to many complimentary educational resources such as her blog, masterclass and podcast, her online clinic provides cutting-edge functional health testing and personalised 1-1 support.

Her first book, It's Not You, It's Your Hormones, has received hundreds of 5* reviews with many claiming it to be an invaluable support for women managing the perimenopausal years.

She is also an ambassador for The Hunger Project, and a supporter of Women For Women International.

INDEX

Symbols

A

B

NRF2 39, 227, 246
Nutrient deficiencies 43, 48, 77, 80, 83, 90, 116, 123, 139, 150, 194, 241
Nutrients :
- Omega-3 Fats 44, 83, 84, 111, 121, 123, 148, 149, 168, 226, 230, 231, 243, 310, 311
- B Vitamins 78, 80, 83, 92, 111, 115, 121, 130, 136, 153, 154, 168, 195, 198, 200, 227, 231, 241, 291, 312
- Vitamin D 18, 37, 44, 79, 80, 93, 103, 106, 111, 112, 115, 121, 129, 130, 135, 143, 158, 159, 160, 168, 187, 197, 198, 200, 202, 226, 241, 242, 250, 262, 265, 310, 311, 312
- Magnesium 78, 79, 80, 81, 90, 93, 103, 106, 108, 112, 115, 122, 157, 158, 160, 165, 167, 169, 195, 200, 215, 227, 235, 241, 242, 301, 311
- Minerals 90, 92, 93, 98, 110, 111, 133, 135, 153, 154, 157, 158, 160, 167, 169, 197, 235, 240, 242, 259, 312
Nutrient Signalling 35, 143
Nuts and Seeds 81, 115, 119, 146, 148, 157, 162, 167

O

Obesity 40, 41, 50, 51, 79, 95, 111, 112, 146, 149, 172, 189, 199, 200, 220, 235, 250, 260, 291, 296, 297, 298, 311
Olive Oil 84, 115, 130, 137, 138, 146, 150, 151, 152, 160, 168, 173, 226, 299
Oxidation, Antioxidants, 38, 39, 43, 44, 150, 151, 227, 242

P

Perimenopause 3, 4, 8, 1, 4, 6, 15, 24, 64, 85, 89, 94, 186, 193, 264
Pesticides 110, 167, 297, 298
Phytoestrogens 92, 108, 117, 123, 163, 165, 166, 231, 243, 258
Phytonutrients, Plant Nutrients 160, 161, 163, 164, 167, 168, 169, 226, 292
Positive Ageing 20, 26, 119
Post Menopause 3, 4, 6, 8, 34, 38, 39, 40, 53, 54, 83, 86, 89, 93, 116, 120, 193, 201, 225, 274, 286, 290, 292
Present Moment 70, 91, 265, 279
Processed Foods 35, 80, 81, 84, 103, 107, 110, 114, 123, 131, 137, 138, 148, 173, 267, 301
Protein 36, 44, 51, 78, 83, 84, 85, 87, 88, 92, 106, 107, 115, 121, 129, 130, 133, 140, 141, 142, 143, 144, 145, 146, 150, 153, 155, 158, 167, 168, 173, 197, 198, 199, 226, 230, 245, 246, 250, 301, 310
Psychoneuroimmunology (PNI) 56
Purpose, Legacy, Contribution 22, 25, 27, 29, 64, 68, 209, 210, 264, 269, 270, 283, 284, 285, 287, 317

R

Red Light Therapy 240, 260
Rest, 7 Types of Rest, Self Care 7, 8, 23, 24, 43, 45, 47, 49, 65, 66, 67, 68, 82, 85, 91, 99, 102, 123, 175, 188, 190, 194, 198, 200, 207, 208, 209, 210, 211, 220, 223, 225, 256, 258, 262, 266, 276, 281, 301

S

Printed in Great Britain
by Amazon